WHAT PEOPLE ARE SAYING ABOUT

WHEN THE ROAD TURNS*...*

"A book that reminds us to hold tight to our dreams, *When the Road Turns* is an inspiring collection of stories written by people living with multiple sclerosis. When you walk through the front door of these writers' lives, you won't leave without a renewed sense of hope and a new definition of courage."

—Montel Williams
entertainer, author and philanthropist

"I was touched by the experiences of faith and hope that these writers express in dealing with MS. I believe that it is not the disease, but the lack of hope that gets one down. These stories champion success in dealing with MS and I am pleased to recommend it."

—Alan Osmond
entertainer, author and founder of One Heart, a nonprofit
organization dedicated to strengthening families

"*When the Road Turns* is filled to overflowing with compelling stories of how to live life to the fullest. It reminds us all of what we are capable of, regardless of what our circumstances might be."

—Olayinka Joseph
author, *Voices of Courage: Everyone Has a Story*

"*When the Road Turns* shows there is life after being diagnosed with multiple sclerosis. This is an amazing, inspirational book. You will come away with a different sense of people and their abilities—not their disabilities."

—Noonie Fortin
author, *Memories of Maggie* and *Potpourri of War*

"Dreams are known as goals with deadlines. *When the Road Turns* is a book that will inspire you to experience your dreams and pursue new ones! It's a masterpiece in motivation. After you read this book, get ready to live your dreams!"

—Steve Kime
professional speaker and author,
How Will They Remember Me?

"Margot Russell has put together a much-needed book. I see the tremendous hope that lives within these words. I am personally encouraged."

—Joanne Wallace
speaker and author, *Starting Over*
and *The Confident Woman*

"Russell's book is a collection of heartwarming and inspirational essays by individuals who have chosen to lead a full life, despite their challenges with MS. Their stories send a clear message: The urging of a person's spirit is a greater power than their disease."

—M. Cathy Angell
author, *My Spirit Flies* and founder of the Power Project

"This is a magnificent book! The strength of the human spirit is expressed in every story. The contributors embrace their challenges with the courage and hope that will inspire anyone who reads this book."

—Karen L. Rose
president, Blooming Rose Seminars
speaker, trainer and author, *Embrace Your Challenging Times:
They Really Are Your Blessings*

WHEN THE ROAD
TURNS

*Inspirational
Stories by and About
People with MS*

M A R G O T   R U S S E L L

Health Communications, Inc.
Deerfield Beach, Florida

www.bci-online.com

Library of Congress Cataloging-in-Publication Data

When the road turns : inspirational stories by and about people with MS / [edited by] Margot Russell.
    p.   cm.
  ISBN 1-55874-907-1 (tradepaper)
  1. Multiple sclerosis—Patients—Biography. I. Russell, Margot, 1962-

RC377 .W48 2001
362.1'96834'0092—dc21
[B]

2001024651

Publisher: Health Communications, Inc.
          3201 S.W. 15th Street
          Deerfield Beach, FL 33442-8190

Cover and inside book design by Lawna Patterson Oldfield
Cover background photos ©PhotoDisc

*This book is dedicated to
all of the people who live with
multiple sclerosis.
And to their families and
loved ones, too.*

CONTENTS

ACKNOWLEDGMENTS

Special thanks to Nowick Gray for dotting the i's and crossing the t's in each of these wonderful stories. Thanks to Dean Kramer for carefully reading each piece and sharing her thoughts and ideas. Thanks to Liz Pendergast for coming up with a list of potential contributors: Many of their stories are included in this book. Thank you Kathleen Wilson at MSWorld for your support and encouragement this past year, and to Paul S. Levine for being a patient and talented agent. Thanks to my editors Allison Janse and Christine Belleris. I also extend my love and thanks to those who contributed to this book by so generously sharing their stories. And loving thanks to my family, especially Bill and my children—Kerry, Colleen and Maggie—for their patience and support.

PROLOGUE

By now you may have heard my story. The first of my MS symptoms appeared when I was in the Naval Academy, I've had recurring bouts every two years, and was misdiagnosed for about twenty years since then. But the details of my diagnosis are not important. What I've done *with* it is.

When I heard the three words "You have MS," like the authors of these stories, I denied, grieved, raged, self-pitied and despaired. I wondered if the fire in my feet would ever go away. I worried that my career and livelihood would be taken from me. I thought about leaving this planet, but couldn't do that to the people who loved me. I sat around for sixty days going "woe is me," but at the end of sixty days, where did that get me? Then a friend said to me, "I don't understand you. You've met every other challenge life has thrown your way. You've moved every other mountain. Why is this one any different?"

The words "You have MS" changed my life, but my friend's words *saved* my life. Because that's when I realized that I've never let anyone or anything define me, define my limits, or take away my hope. And I wasn't about to let MS.

That's what I like about these stories. MS doesn't define these authors; they define MS. They are not waiting around for MS to beat them; they are working, living, playing and beating MS. Each of them has discovered that switch in their minds that turned them from MS sufferers to MS survivors. The day I found that switch was the day I realized, I have MS; *it doesn't have me.*

One of my favorite adages is "What have I done today that's worth talking about tomorrow?" What each of these authors has accomplished is worth talking about. They remind me of a favorite quote from Anne Frank: "Whoever is happy will make others happy, too. He who has courage and faith will never perish in misery."

Montel Williams
entertainer, author and founder of
The Montel Williams MS Foundation

FOREWORD

It is hard to sum up a book in one word, but if I had to choose one to describe this volume, it would be "journey." This book describes the journey called multiple sclerosis (MS), as it is taken by a number of remarkable people. The journey was not one any of the contributors to this book planned to take. They were plucked unexpectedly out of their everyday lives and propelled in directions they never anticipated. What sorts of journeys were these, and what did they find along the way?

To a great extent, they discovered that multiple sclerosis is a journey inward, and what they ultimately found on this journey was a new identity. This rebirth, this reinventing of the self in response to MS, is described in each chapter. Confronted with uncertainty, pain, physical limitations, financial reverse and social upheaval, all worked to build new identities while remaining true to themselves. And while they often had help from others in the course of their journeys, in essence, each experienced a very personal and individual process.

MS can cause tragic disruption in the best of lives, and none of the authors attempted to minimize the dark significance of this chronic disabling illness. However, in each story we see unfolding the extraordinary ways in which people respond to the challenges of MS. While dealing with many negatives, all managed to accumulate a wealth of positive experiences by drawing upon their own inner resources. In many cases, the extent of these resources came as a surprise, like a magnificent vista that bursts into view when you turn a corner during a journey through unfamiliar territory.

MS challenges different people in different ways, and these stories testify to the amazing variety of coping strategies used to meet those challenges. The stories also reveal many common experiences and themes. The fear and uncertainty aroused by those first symptoms of MS are almost inevitably confronted with denial. Denial and reluctance to deal directly with the illness often leave family and friends feeling shut out. Paradoxically, MS forced many to examine and then bid farewell to comfortable habits of passivity: it became "push ahead or be left behind." Determination and persistence were defining qualities that made the seemingly impossible possible. And through it all, what kept most people going, was the fact that they pursued their dreams of where they wanted to go and who they wanted to be. As readers, we are fortunate to be able to share some of these dreams and the kaleidoscope of emotions experienced by the authors.

I started out by saying that these were stories by and about remarkable people. However, the real lesson of this book is that under certain conditions perfectly ordinary people can and do accomplish extraordinary things. It is hard to write about a book like this without stumbling over clichés such as "tragic disease," "heroic story" and "courageous fight," but we see these and more in the illuminating pages of this very personal and intimate book. When you are finished reading this book, you will feel as if you have gotten to know several new friends. The reading will fill you with hope that you, too, with all your imperfections and limitations, can accomplish extraordinary things. With the right dream, there is no telling where life's journey can lead.

Nicholas LaRocca, Ph.D.

NICHOLAS LAROCCA *is a clinical psychologist who since 1979 has been working with people who have MS. He is the former Director of Research at the Medical Rehabilitation Research and Training Center for Multiple Sclerosis at St. Agnes Hospital, White Plains, New York, and Associate Professor of Neurology and Medicine at New York Medical College. He recently became Director of Health Care Delivery and Policy Research at the National Multiple Sclerosis Society in New York City.*

INTRODUCTION

Where were you when the road turned? Had you just set out with compass in hand, a map of the miles you would travel in your pocket, feet tapping lightly as you slowly made your way?

Perhaps you were resting along the distant hilltops of your hopes. You had learned to grow roses, had bought a house, had begun to paint. Your business had grown along with your children, and now that you were somewhere there was nowhere left to go.

Until the road turned.

It turned, as it will sometimes, not with a slow and gentle curve, but with decided direction, off to the east, off to the west. No time now to draw another map or pack a different bag. You found your life suddenly defined by circumstance rather than the motion of your feet.

What any person does in the face of adversity is the stuff of which life is made. It is clear that our meaning is not measured by its lack of change, but by its willingness to change. We evolve, marking the years by our growth, our failures and triumphs, by the paths we choose to walk and the ones that we do not.

Perhaps we are most defined in moments of adversity, when we are called upon to be fully human, to embrace the unknown and accept its outcomes, to determine who we are by the choices we make in the heart of uncertainty. Our growth depends not on finding the easiest path to the end of the road, but on accepting the road itself for whatever it brings. We learn from its every twist, embracing what is contrary for all that it can teach us, accepting the opposite of what seems good and just so that we may understand more fully what joy is.

Many people have come to see disease as a gift in their lives. They've found that somewhere along the way they began to view things differently: Routine activities have taken on a richer hue. They've delighted in seeing their child walk through the door. Baking bread, going to work or planting a tree has become a sacred task. They began to live in the moment, as if each and every second were a true gift: Returning to their gardens, they have dug through the dirt and found their roots.

Certainly, facing disease is not the only way to enlightenment, but for those who do not live with a full sense of awareness, it is one way. Often those with an illness learn that they are more than their disease, and once freed by that certainty, they go on to live the rest of the story. They learn a different song, find a shorter route, trade in one costume for another. Poking through life's bag of magic tricks, they find that recreating themselves has always been a possibility.

When the road turned for me, the hardest issue was acceptance. I wasn't prepared for a disease whose very essence seemed to demand the best of me, whose presence suggested my future was not my own to decide. I mourned the shortened list of possibilities for myself. I wasn't willing to adapt.

I began to communicate with and observe the many others who seemed to be paddling along beside me. I was inspired by their stories, and often bewildered by their perseverance. I came to see the differences between what I had thought about multiple sclerosis and what I observed.

The first myth I managed to dispel was that everyone with MS would find herself in a wheelchair. While certainly that fact brought relief, much later I found out that I had missed the point. My job in this process was to learn to see myself as a viable person no matter what the outcome, no matter what disabilities I might have to endure.

Writing about multiple sclerosis is difficult; the disease varies from person to person, and what is true for one may not be true for another. While we may applaud one person with MS for sailing across the Atlantic or running a marathon, in the next breath we must applaud the person with a progressive case for being able to walk again after a particularly bad episode. We must applaud the mother in a wheelchair for the kind and loving care she is able to give to her children; we must praise the newly diagnosed father who makes his way to work.

This book is a compilation of stories from people who found themselves at a crossroad. When their roads turned, they were forced to throw away their maps and take a different route. What they realized along the way was that they were *not* their experience; rather, their lives were newly created by what they *made* of their experience.

The people who contributed to this book are inspirations. I hope they will continue to change the face of multiple sclerosis by teaching us that there is a world beyond the disease, that we can leave behind our baggage and make our way again.

There is value to be found in every life, no matter what limitations or boundaries are imposed. When we are willing to change our expectations, we are free to appreciate the essence of who we really are.

Where were you when the road turned?

And, now, where will you go?

Margot Russell
January 5, 2000

*It is not our purpose to become each other;
it is to recognize each other, to learn
to see the other and honor
him for what he is.*

HERMANN HESSE

1

DENIAL

Barbara Sullivan Roehrig

I only told a half dozen friends that I had been diagnosed with multiple sclerosis. I asked my family not to share the news with anyone until I had coped with it myself.

Unfortunately, my mother chose to make it her own telemarketing campaign, because now *she* had a daughter with MS. So, I had to answer telephone calls from people I hadn't seen or heard from since high school.

At that time, I was merely trying to stick my big toe into the waters of chronic disease. I wanted to see how it felt first. But the callers were under the impression that my life was in great peril and that I was terribly sick. Responding to their concerns was not what I wanted to do just then, so this marked the beginning of my "denial campaign," when I exclaimed to the callers, "Oh, I'm feeling on top of the world!"

I truly believed that I was going to be one of the many people with MS in the relapsing-remitting stage, and that I would never have another flare-up for the rest of my life.

> I FIND IT INTERESTING TO SEE HOW AT EASE I WAS PRETENDING TO BE SOMEONE ELSE WITH MS: JUST AS LONG AS IT WASN'T ME.

When a film producer asked if I would appear in an HBO documentary on chronic disease, I explained that I was nowhere near ready to "come out" on national television. It was a couple of years after my diagnosis, yet half of my close friends didn't even know I had MS. So I told him I would be happy to work behind the scenes and provide all of the background information they needed, but I didn't want to appear on camera. I encouraged him to scout for talent elsewhere.

Months later, he called back, explaining that he had scoured the country for potential candidates, but still felt I was the perfect person to appear in the documentary. I resisted once again. But in his determination to have me on camera, he convinced me to appear in disguise—as a red-head with short hair, lots of make-up and a fictitious name.

Surely, I thought, no one would be able to recognize me. I had long, naturally curly brown hair and I hardly ever wore make-up.

Until then, I hadn't focused on my illness for more than an hour at a time, so the three days that I filmed with the crew were excruciatingly painful. At the same time, since I was wearing a disguise, I was able to appear fairly comfortable being filmed. The crew wanted to capture someone coping with a chronic disease on a daily basis. Looking back, I find it interesting to see how at ease I was pretending to be someone else with MS: just as long as it wasn't me.

I was in therapy at the time, learning how to cope with the sudden change in my health, so the camera crew sat in on my therapy session that week. I'm sure they were as stunned as my therapist as I described an experience I had suffered through the weekend before.

The camera crew taped my every word as I explained my philosophy about wellness to my therapist: "I'll try anything once. It may work!" With this in mind, I said I had attended a special service heralded as a "healing session" at my Catholic church. I found myself, that beautiful Saturday afternoon, sitting in the pews among the ill and the hopeful. I listened attentively to the lecturer, as if my strong intention and motivation to heal would facilitate the process.

The healer spoke of cancers, skin disorders and a host of other illnesses. Then, after a dramatic pause, he spoke of "the dreadful diseases," which, among others, included multiple sclerosis.

I have a dreadful disease? What does that mean? I wondered. Weren't the other diseases he mentioned just as dreadful? And what is the distinction between a regular disease and a dreadful disease?

I felt crippled by the drama of his rhetoric. He had blown the wind right out of my sails. I had come to the session for healing, but I felt like I was dealt a knockout punch in a title bout.

I decided not to walk out, though. Something inside of me still wanted to believe that I would be healed: I wasn't going to endure his caustic words without realizing some benefit from them. So I went through the process of waving my arms, shouting out loud, holding hands with the faithful and praying.

The cameras continued to roll as I ended this story in my therapist's office. I sobbed as I remembered every painful moment. "This was supposed to be healing?" I asked. "I guess it hasn't happened yet—it must be a healing process with a long shelf life. It's going to kick in any day now!"

Over the next few days, the cameras followed me everywhere. They went with me to the airport, to physical therapy, to the Denver Museum of Nature and Science and to my neurology appointment—which seemed to amuse my neurologist. I explained beforehand that there'd be cameras following me into the office, and I requested that she call me "Gail" instead of Barbara. When I mentioned that I'd be in disguise, she said, "Great! Can they make me thin, beautiful and six feet tall?"

When the filming ended, I was physically and emotionally drained. It hadn't been easy sharing so much of myself with relative strangers. But the director of the documentary assured me that my participation was sure to positively impact others coping with a chronic disease. We had a bite to eat together before he left; he promised to forward any letters that came in after the documentary was aired, and he said he'd keep in touch.

When he failed to keep in touch, I tried to contact him several times over the next few months. I usually reached his producer, who was suddenly much more accessible to me than her boss. "How is the filming going?" I'd ask. "How about the editing? What does HBO think of your work?" Intuitively, I felt like I was being pushed away.

Finally, the director returned one of my many phone calls. "Your scenes were cut," he said. "The double identity just didn't work. It wasn't real enough to have you in disguise."

I was devastated—all of this for naught? It would take me years to finally understand the pearl that was given to me: A double identity doesn't work.

Finding the "real me" was a slow process. Making the

transition from a state of denial to being truthful with others about my disease was the equivalent of turning the *Queen Mary*. For a long time, I didn't tell any of my coworkers or business associates about my illness. Then, as the years passed and the disease progressed, I started hobbling off airplanes with a cane. I had been hiding my condition, and now it was readily apparent to any onlooker.

A big turning point for me was a televised speech that I gave for the Heuga Center at the Snow Mountain Express event on Copper Mountain in the winter of 1999. The Heuga Center holds five-day personal fitness programs and emotional well-being sessions tailored to people with multiple sclerosis. I had attended a session a few years before and was very impressed by the program. When the center holds sporting events to raise funds, a past participant is usually invited to talk about his or her experiences. More than one hundred people were watching in the audience, and a hush fell over the room as I began my speech.

I thought I seemed like a babbling idiot as I related my experiences of the program, how life-changing it had been for me and how the center encourages everyone to be the absolute best that they can be, no matter what that "best" might look like.

When the speech ended, I realized I had gained strength from disclosing my disease, by being honest and frank. I had feared people would pity me, but I later learned that many in the audience had been very moved by my words. It had never occurred to me that I could inspire others by living a full life despite having a challenging illness.

Another turning point was my participation in a three-day, self-defense workshop designed for women. That experience—a woman who walks with such difficulty knocking out multiple assailants—was mind-blowing. I cried the first night when we told each other why we were there. I cried during graduation. There is great assurance in knowing that I can take care of myself, even with my physical shortcomings, even when traveling alone on business.

Bit by bit, slowly but surely, I have become more comfortable with the real me. And it seems that the more I disclose to others, the more I am supported, both emotionally and physically.

I recently spoke at a conference in my capacity as a marketing consultant for a large cable company. A man leaned over while I was checking voice mails on the pay phone and asked me why I had a cane. I calmly and confidently said, "Oh, I have MS." He immediately explained that he knew many people with MS; we instantly connected.

More recently, while speaking at a business conference, a gentleman complimented me on the cane I was carrying. I thanked him and told him about the woman from Boston who has MS and makes the canes herself. He asked if I'd had an injury; I explained that I had MS.

He then told me that his father had become a double amputee suddenly, and he described the struggles his father had endured as a result.

I now recognize the beautiful dynamic that results when a person shares something with another person. That "something" may be a truth, or a raw and vulnerable wound that heals a little more each time it's shared. When the person on the other end receives the pearl, he or she often reciprocates by sharing something personal. As a result, the two are forever connected in some way by the sometimes brief, but meaningful, exchange.

My decision to accept and even relish whatever comes my way is mine, and mine alone, to make. The way I look at it, my attitude is one of the few things that I can completely control in life—and I intend to do just that. I now freely tell people that I have MS, and my spirit feels a little stronger each time I do.

BARBARA SULLIVAN ROEHRIG *lives in Denver, Colorado, with her husband, Chip Roehrig. She runs her own market- ing consulting firm out of her home and serves clients in the high-tech industry domestically and worldwide. She is actively involved as a board member of Adventures Within, and is a volunteer for organizations as varied as the Heuga Center, the Colorado Symphony Orchestra and Boston College Club of Colorado.*

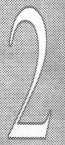

MOVING TOWARD ACCEPTANCE

Gary Shane Lavenson

This is the story of my own miracle. I set off for Greece to participate in an experimental treatment for multiple sclerosis, hoping to find a cure. Impossible, maybe, but what I learned along the way was an even greater gift.

When I found out in 1985 that I had multiple sclerosis, I began a relentless search for relief from my condition. All of my friends and family were concerned, but no one knew what to do. They seemed to have an endless supply of suggestions and advice, countless articles and books and medical reports. Everyone had a story about someone or something that could cure me. They blamed my condition on bad diet, bad water, environmental hazards or mercury poisoning from the fillings in my teeth.

I was nineteen years old when the symptoms first started. A small dot appeared in my visual field and became a part of the landscape. Four months later, it disappeared, but not forever. When I was thirty-one, it returned like a long-lost friend and brought with it a host of other symptoms.

> I WAS NEVER ABLE TO PLAY SOCCER WITH [MY SON], BUT . . . I THINK HE KNOWS THAT THE PART OF ME STRUGGLING TO GET WELL IS THE PART THAT LOVES HIM MOST.

Now that my symptoms were more pervasive than a single bouncing dot, my doctors were certain that I had MS. At the age of thirty-one—husband, musician, athlete, father—I was diagnosed with a disease for which there is no cure.

I had spent much of my adult life engaged in physical activity. Performing in my band, I'd prance around the stage like Bruce Springsteen and be the last to leave the party. In the mornings, I rushed off to my job as a real estate agent.

In my free time, I'd take long walks in the mountains of New Hampshire and camp with my family. I loved the outdoors: horseback riding, scuba diving and hiking. MS would one day take these activities and turn them into ancient dreams.

The relationships that I valued most began to change after my diagnosis. My daughter, who was three at the time, wanted to run around the yard with me and ride bikes like we always had. It was hard to explain the fatigue to her or the weakness in my legs. As for my son, he was born a year after I was diagnosed. He'd never remember the days when I was strong enough to lift him, play ball with him or run.

My marriage was already showing strain in the days before I was diagnosed, and the complications that my health brought to our lives seemed to widen the cracks. I was resentful of my wife's attitude toward my disease, which seemed to fluctuate between defeat and unrestrained acceptance. At one point, she asked her father to build a wheelchair ramp around the house to prepare for what she thought was the inevitable outcome of my life. I wasn't quite ready to throw in the towel, but she felt she was being sensitive.

MS can bring havoc to one's sexual life, and mine was no exception. Sexual dysfunction isn't an easy thing to talk about, and my wife and I seemed to lack the skills to communicate with each other about intimacy.

I also began to sense a division in attitude toward my disease. It seemed some people were sympathetic, while others were resentful. This division is understandable because sometimes I would appear as if nothing were wrong and other times I could barely stand up. No one knew what to expect. Some people thought I was faking it. "You certainly look fine," they would say while shaking their heads. Some believed that I had brought it on myself. I mulled over the possibility of karma and past sins.

I have left no stone unturned when it comes to treatments and remedies for MS. I've been given steroids to help deal with the pain and the loss of mobility. I've experimented with health-food diets such as macrobiotics. I've tried megavitamins, meditation, acupuncture and chiropractors. I've consulted faith healers, psychics and medical dowsers, and I've attended MS support groups. I've had appointments with neurologists and research specialists. I've even been to the Ayurvedic clinic to see Deepak Chopra, the spiritual leader and writer. I have found relief from time to time in doing all these things, but I think that most of the benefit has come from the efforts I made on my own behalf. After all of this, I have come to view multiple sclerosis as a divine mystery.

In July 1992, my brother Michael sent me an article from the *Washington Post* that described an amazing new treatment for MS. Miraculous results were reported for some MS patients who were stung by honeybees ten to thirty times every other day. Claims of phenomenal improvement and even cure were presented. All one had to do was withstand multiple bee stings.

I started with six stings every other day and gradually built up to ten, and then twenty. People who witnessed me getting stung found it hard to believe their eyes; most people could not even watch. I'd grab the buzzing bee with a pair of extra-long surgical tweezers, set it on my arm, close my eyes and within seconds I'd be stung. It was painful, yet I welcomed it. The potential benefits certainly outweighed the three or four seconds of suffering as the bee sank its stinger into my skin.

At first, the results were spectacular. To the astonishment of my friends and family, I immediately put down my cane and walked up and down stairs.

I, too, was surprised by these results, but my success didn't last very long. Soon I experienced only fifteen minutes of relief after each sting. The treatment had been absolutely free for me, and only the little honeybee had paid—with its life.

When a new drug treatment called interferon therapy came out, I stopped the bee stings and learned to use a hypodermic needle. This was the newest treatment for MS, and its release into the MS community was followed by quite a bit of fanfare. So, I injected myself every other day with this $10,000-a-year drug, sticking with it for at least six months, but in the end the side effects became unbearable. I decided there had to be something better, but I never dreamed where my search would take me.

❖ ❖ ❖ ❖

When I told everyone I was going to Greece for an experimental MS treatment, everyone warned me not to go. One friend asked, "When was the last time you heard of a great doctor from Greece?" As for my doctor, he shook his head: "You could find yourself there, having complications from the chemotherapy. And then what? What would we do? We couldn't exactly send an ambulance!"

I heard all kinds of misgivings about going to Athens for an unfamiliar, low-level chemotherapy treatment administered by an unknown doctor, but I was driven by the need to get well. My instincts told me to go, so I started planning.

Except for driving to Canada, vacationing in the Virgin Islands and once walking across the border into Mexico, I had never left the United States. I certainly had never entertained the thought of going to another country in search of a miracle cure.

My decision seemed punctuated by little signs and coincidences. When I had finally found the phone number for the doctor in Athens and called him, the doctor himself answered. It was far easier to reach him than it was my own doctor in the States! I began to wonder if it was some kind of scam, until I remembered that I had called him. I thought it too unlikely that he had been sitting by the phone waiting for the next sucker to call. No, I felt, I had just stumbled onto something incredible.

As the plane made its way to Athens, I thought of my wife and children. When we had said our good-byes in the morning, I had tried to reassure them. "I'll be back before you know it," I said, "and, hopefully, I'll be walking like a new man!" I told my son Jamie I'd yell his name from a mountaintop in Greece so loud that he could hear me all the way in America. The thought seemed to comfort him.

As soon as I landed, I got into my own collapsible wheelchair and was escorted into a Mercedes cab. That was the way my trip to Athens started, with Costas, my first new friend and cab driver.

Costas was an unbelievably energetic and bright face in my dark and unknown future. A ball of energy with a laugh like a roar, he was also a charming con artist. With his styled jet-black hair and million-dollar smile, he looked more like a soap opera star than a taxi driver.

When I first got in the cab, we eyeballed each other. It was obvious he didn't speak English very well, so I asked him a very simple question: "Do you like American music?"

His face lit up. "Rock and roll?" he asked.

I had brought some musical items with me to help break the ice. I had several CDs containing my own songs, some Silvertone harmonicas, my Vagabond travel guitar and various cassette tapes.

"Yes! Rock and roll!" I replied with fervor. I immediately pulled one of the Silvertone harmonicas out of my pocket and played a few blues riffs for him. His eyes lit up again, and I asked if he liked the blues.

"Yes, I like blues, like blues much!" he said in his broken English. I handed him my harp and told him to try it. I guess he thought I was giving it to him, because he slipped it into his pocket as we were talking.

My internal camera jumped to an aerial view, and I saw myself for a moment in the backseat of Costas's Mercedes taxi, racing down the highway. I felt a rush of emotion as I realized I was actually in Athens, Greece, heading to Dr. Kountouris's office to begin a treatment that might cure my condition.

I hadn't seen anything likable about Greece yet, mostly concrete buildings and clothes stores. I strained to see something remarkable and caught a glimpse of the Parthenon in the distance. Costas was entertaining me with his wild stories, his positive attitude and the energy he put into finding the right English words to express himself.

It was easy to forget about my long history of bodily malfunction, while I was getting to know my new friend. I was thirty-one when I was officially diagnosed with multiple sclerosis. Over the years, I have been confronted with a wide variety of challenging disabilities.

Most of my symptoms are typical of MS: bowel and bladder problems, fatigue and weakness. I've had speech problems, and I've sometimes lost the ability to perform simple daily functions. I've had shooting, debilitating pain in my legs and abdomen. At times, the pain was so intense that I would wake up screaming at night, begging God to spare me.

One time I became paralyzed from the neck down for two months. I was told that I would probably never walk again. Thank God they were wrong about that, but there are still long periods when I need a cane just to make it to my car. Sometimes I am so weak that I cannot make it to the kitchen.

The most profound discovery I have made is that a placebo might be just as effective as actual medicine 60 percent of the time. Sometimes it is hard to judge where the benefit to one's well-being is coming from. Perhaps a spiritual experience can facilitate physical healing. Perhaps one's frame of mind is inexplicably connected to one's health.

I had learned to put great faith in the power of my own beliefs, an idea I had cultivated by reading spiritual healing books. Perhaps, I thought, this is all that medicine is: an elixir whose power to heal is determined by our thoughts about it. I was beginning to think that nothing was impossible, as long as we believed.

Costas took me to my hotel and helped me with my luggage. He gave me his home phone and cellular numbers, and told me to call if I needed anything at all.

I gave him one of the CDs, which seemed to thrill him, and said good-bye. I never thought I would see him again.

Alone in front of the hotel, my thoughts turned to Dr. Kountouris and the chemotherapy treatment. The words "I believe, I believe" were chanting in my head.

My first appointment with Dr. Kountouris was scheduled for the next day. I was planning on taking things very slowly. I even contemplated not taking the treatment at all until I was comfortable and had talked to other patients. I wanted to become familiar with the doctor and his protocol. I didn't think anyone would blame me for turning around and coming home if the treatment appeared to be hazardous to my health.

I awoke with anticipation in the morning. Today I would meet the man who claimed to have the newest, most highly effective treatment for multiple sclerosis—a man I knew of only from a small article someone had found in a newspaper.

According to the article, the treatment involved the use of a chemotherapy drug called mitoxantrone. Mitoxantrone was used in the United States to treat prostate cancer and a form of leukemia, but had never been used to treat MS. "No side effects," the article had claimed, because it was given in small doses.

I had asked my own doctor if he had heard of the treatment. He hadn't and said he had no interest in finding out more about it. If it was something worthy, he felt he would hear about it through the normal channels. The fact that I had discovered it in a newspaper impressed him even less.

My doctor had spent the last four or five years trying to convince me to start cytoxan and metheltrexate, which are chemotherapy treatments approved for targeting MS. Both were reputed to have very strong side effects. I had avoided his advice, because I was afraid to consider anything as invasive as traditional chemotherapy. I was more encouraged about Dr. Kountouris's treatment because he claimed there were no side effects at all when mitoxantrone was given in low dosages with immunoglobulins. Finding no help from my doctor, I had called the Multiple Sclerosis Society and was told that they, too, were trying to locate Dr. Kountouris. They were actively searching the Internet and would know more the next week. The society's phone was ringing off the hook with people looking for information.

I decided to call the Reuters News Agency in Athens, the source of the newspaper article. The person who answered the phone told me that he was an eyewitness to people being wheeled into the doctor's office and then actually walking out by the end of an eighteen-month period. I liked the sound of that. He also claimed that Dr. Kountouris had more than one thousand patients. Then he gave me the phone number for the reporter who actually wrote the article, who in turn gave me the number of the doctor's office. This is how I became the first American pioneer to make contact with Dr. Dimitris Kountouris. Or perhaps, I considered, I was the first fool!

Dr. D. himself had answered the phone when I first called from the States. He seemed to speak English well enough. He had me fax my medical history to him and then replied immediately, saying that he thought he could help me but I would have to come to Athens for the treatment. He explained that I would stay for two months and then continue the treatment at home. The price would be 500,000 drachmas, or $2,400, which seemed reasonable to me.

Just after noon, I wheeled myself the one block to the doctor's office. Anastasia, the office administrator, welcomed me in fluent English. I was happy to find she was expecting me. Beaming with encouragement, she introduced me to Dr. Kountouris as he came into the room. We shook hands. "Crazy American," he said with a warmhearted smile. I think he was amazed I was there.

The doctor was busy giving orders to the people around him as he glided through the rooms of his clinic, yet in just a few seconds, he had made me feel welcome and at ease. We had immediately established a mutual closeness and trust, a meeting of the minds. Without saying very much, I felt we both knew what we wanted and expected.

He asked me to walk without my cane, but I could not.

He evaluated my situation as I hobbled around the tables and the nurses who were watching with him. Then he said, "Okay, sit!" and was off to another patient.

I definitely had the feeling that I was in the right place. Amazed at how many MS patients were there, all my fears began to dissipate. I really dropped my guard when I started talking to some English-speaking patients. They explained to me how good they were feeling since starting the treatment.

Next, two nurses took a blood sample, along with my blood pressure. They hooked me up to an intravenous fluid bag. I remember feeling a rush of panic when the first needle plunged into my veins. A clear liquid began dripping down from the bottle above. My mind raced and reeled. It was a terrifying, invasive feeling, and I turned my head so that I couldn't see. I had no idea that I would be getting an IV twice a day until my departure on December 13, and that my arms would become totally black and blue.

Fifteen to twenty patients in two rooms were receiving IVs. Some were sitting, others were lying down. Doctor Kountouris came over to where I was lying and praised me for being brave enough to come all the way from America for his treatment. "Crazy American!" he said again with a smile. "You will go home a champion!"

The doctor was a big man with a wave of black hair sporting a distinctive gray streak in the front. He was fairly young, about forty-five years old, and incredibly overworked. He had tremendous pressure on him to give answers and be everywhere at once. People were coming at him from every direction. The phone was ringing constantly. Nurses were being given instructions. Patients were coming and going, and men were making deliveries. Quite a hustle and bustle pervaded the office. I wasn't saying much, but found comfort in the fact that I had seen thirty or more MS patients come and go since my arrival.

Dr. Kountouris introduced me to Theo, the physical therapist. While the IV continued to drip into my vein, Theo began testing my legs and spent fifty minutes bending and stretching them, trying to determine their strength and range of flexibility. Next, he hooked me up to an electronic stimulus machine that zapped me with a low-voltage charge for an hour. He began by hooking two wires to each leg below the knee and sending a charge of electricity through them, gradually increasing the voltage to determine my threshold of pain. At first I was afraid. The language barrier didn't allow me to ask questions, and I felt like a specimen in a strange laboratory project. Each time Theo increased the voltage, the muscles in my legs contracted and the skin beneath the wires received a jolt of radiating heat. It took ten minutes to get used to the treatment, and indeed, weeks later it became a normal and predictable part of the day.

Theo and Dr. Kountouris spoke in Greek, which of course, I could not understand. "You are very easy case for me," said Dr. D. as he turned to me. "You will be my prize when you go back to America!" Then he gave me a peace sign and shouted, "Yankee, go home! No more war! Yankee go home!" I suppose Dr. D. was trying to show me he was from my generation by making a reference to the Vietnam War.

I have always had a hard time trusting doctors unless they are older and wiser than I am. But I had no trouble trusting Dr. D. I only had trouble speaking with him, unless I used the universal language of rock 'n' roll. When I asked him if he liked American music, he strummed his air guitar and sang, "Give me a ticket for an air-o-plane."

In the company of this likable doctor, I fantasized what it would be like to ski again, climb mountains or play ball with my kids. Maybe I would dance with my wife again. I wondered why I trusted this crazy Greek. Only when I thought about my other options did I appreciate once more why I was here.

Before I left Dr. Kountouris's office the first day, I was introduced to Marina Angeli, the psychiatrist, psychotherapist and flower therapist. The doctor yelled to her, as he was walking away, "No alternative stuff for him!" I was intrigued and asked her what he meant. "My flower therapy," she explained, "it is not for everyone." She promised to explain the next day when we would have more time.

I wheeled myself back to my hotel that afternoon and left the wheelchair behind the stairwell. I wouldn't need it again until I left Athens, almost six weeks later.

❖ ❖ ❖ ❖

When I returned to the doctor's office the next day, I met with Marina Angeli. She had a very calm and warmhearted approach, and she spoke English very well. I found myself taking advantage of her psychotherapy skills and immediately started confiding in her. I think because she spoke such fluent English and because I hadn't had anyone to converse with, I expressed all my fears and anxieties.

I told her about my father and my feelings of abandonment. I told her about my marital and sexual problems. Everything flowed out of me like a waterfall and I started to cry. I thought she would solve all of my problems with a wave of her hand. I chuckle now when I remember how she simply acknowledged me, and then presented me with a bottle of flower essences.

"Here," she said, handing me a little bottle marked "Bach Flowers." "This is what you need. Try it for two weeks. It should help you adjust to your new environment. It will also help you with your confidence and self-esteem." I marveled at the little bottle. She told me to put four drops on my tongue. It was actually delicious.

It did seem to help me with my self-esteem and confidence, just as she said it would. It wasn't just the bit of brandy mixed into the bottle; there was something else good about it. I liked taking it out of my pocket when I needed to bolster my oomph or build up my pizzazz. I really can't explain why, but I know I needed Marina Angeli and the magic of her flower therapy to get me through the next eight weeks.

I was feeling very happy that I had made the decision to come to Athens. The large number of MS patients at the clinic encouraged me. I liked Dr. Kountouris and his staff. I liked what was in those IV bottles. And whatever Theo and Marina were doing, it was working. I guess you could say I was off to a good start.

After my second treatment one day, I was feeling so good that I asked Theo to let me take him to dinner. The trouble was, Theo wasn't the type who liked to go out to dinner. (Dr. Kountouris called him a communist. He called himself a socialist and me an imperialist). I know Theo's type. He doesn't like going out to eat because he hates to spend the money—even if it isn't his—and because he can cook so much better himself.

For some reason, Theo accepted my invitation and ordered grilled fish at the restaurant. I was amazed at his delight in eating the whole thing, head and all. He also loved wine, and he had no trouble finishing the whole bottle. By the end of the meal, he had become quite animated and was making great fun of the American medical world.

Theo viewed my disease as if it were no big deal. I was simply disabled and nothing more. I only needed to build up my confidence and get rid of my fears, and then I could have a productive life. I liked his matter-of-fact thinking. I wanted to believe in this simple approach to healing. I did not fully realize, that evening, how important Theo would become to me, as there came a day when he may have actually saved my life.

When I experience fatigue, I usually try to do little more than wait for my energy to return. I am never really sure where the energy comes from when it does come back. Sometimes I try to will it back; other times I try to take the right vitamins or exercise in a certain way. I have come up with dozens of methods, and I sometimes think that I have found the one that works.

Theo believes it is our attitudes that make the difference. He would always tell me that my mind was strong, but my heart was weak. He'd say, "You think you can't walk, but you can." Those words would play over and over in my head.

After an hour of therapy, Theo would come over and take my cane away. "Now, walk!" he would say. Though I didn't know how, I would. I realized that I had to believe it was possible first, but where do you drum up that faith?

Theo and the mighty Dr. D. were somewhat insulting at times. Perhaps it was an effort on their part to snap me out of self-pity. I would hobble over to their office, feeling very tired, and they would say, "Tired? Why tired? Why always tired?"

"Because I am," I would say.

"No!" Theo would shout. "You not tired! You scared!"

I had trouble arguing. It felt like tired to me.

After some noticeable improvement the first week, I thought I had found a miracle cure by the second week. I felt so good after all of my twice-daily, ninety-minute treatments that I would get up and walk with confidence, moving almost like a normal man.

It was hard to say if it was the drugs administered by Dr. D. or the physical therapy that had the most effect. I gave a lot of credit to the work that Theo did with his electronic stimulus, laser beams, heat lamps and strange suction device. Clearly, this wasn't the traditional physical therapy that is used in the States, but I thought surely I'd found my dream team.

After three weeks I was feeling so much stronger that Dr. Kountouris came up to me and said, "By this weekend, you must play soccer!" He knew that I had promised to play soccer with my son when I returned home.

"You must be ready!" he said. "You must be great! Now show me your walk!" He demonstrated how he wanted me to walk, with big steps. *"Migalo vima,* Gary, *migalo vima!"*

I liked the sound of the words "big step" in Greek. First he said *"migalo"* and I would take a step. Then he'd say *"vima"* and I would take another.

I was feeling good and walking well, and I delighted in showing off. I was walking without my cane while Theo and the other patients looked on, shouting "Bravo! Bravo!"

I loved the sound of that word too. When I walked by at a brisk pace with my cane, even some of the shop-keepers on Michalakopoulou Street came out of their stores and yelled, "Bravo! Bravo!" What would they say now? I could hear the cheers already.

I felt wonderful after my treatment and went down-stairs to Othello's Restaurant for a salad and steak. As I got up to leave, I realized that I had lost strength.

The walk back to the hotel seemed like a million miles. I was leaning heavily upon my cane. I couldn't believe that I had felt so good one minute, yet needed my cane the next to walk. I struggled very slowly down the street.

Migalo vima. Migalo vima.

Cars and scooters rushed by.

Migalo vima. Each step was a struggle.

And then I fell in the streets of Athens.

Cars screeched to a halt. A man jumped out of his car and came to where I was lying. I struggled to stand on my own, but decided it felt better to lie back down.

I lay there listening to the hustle and bustle of traffic resuming. I felt myself almost drifting off to sleep until two men began lifting me up from each side. *"Efcharisto,"* I blurted out in my best Greek. "Thank you."

"Why fall?" the man on my right asked.

"These stupid shoes," I said, walking away with a wobble.

It became a day-to-day routine. I arrived at 10:00 or 11:00 in the morning and received two or three bottles of IV infusion. Then I would walk across the street to Theo's for physical therapy. Then it was back to my hotel for a nap. I would return at 7:00 or 8:00 P.M. for another IV infusion, and then go back to Theo's by 8:00 for another round of physical therapy.

I had some moments of incredible strength and exhilaration during the treatments. Those were the moments that I wanted to share with everyone. I would fax my family and write to my friends. I kept thinking how wonderful it would be to go back home on my own two feet and not in my wheelchair.

I decided to trade in my wheelchair for a bicycle. What a wonderful thought! It would be a great headline for an MS newsletter: "Man Arrives in Greece with Wheelchair and Leaves on Bicycle." I phoned my mother and whispered, "Mom, don't tell anyone. I'm going to trade in my wheelchair for a bicycle." I wanted her to be the first to know the incredible news before it hit the newspapers.

My mother hung up the phone and immediately called the rest of the family. She told them that I was undoubtedly on some kind of mind-altering drug.

At 5:00 A.M. on December 10, close to the end of my stay in Athens, I woke up in my hotel room and realized that I was shaking with fever. I tried to move and felt panic surge through my body. I could only move my head and arms. The rest of my body was paralyzed. I couldn't even sit up to pull the covers off my legs.

"Don't panic," I told myself.

I couldn't reach the phone; it was two feet too far away. I decided to go back to sleep, but I awoke again an hour later. I still had the shakes and a very high fever. I wanted to cool down the room, but I couldn't move. I was terrified.

With great effort, I managed to pull the phone over to me so that I could call the front desk. I told them to send someone up to open my windows and bring me some bottled water.

I lay there hearing the words of my doctor back home: "You could be over there and have complications from the chemo. Then what would we do?" I struggled to keep myself calm. I didn't want my journey to Athens to end on such a bad note. Finally, two maids came into my room, and I asked them to help me sit up. I felt like a beached whale as they grabbed my arms on either side and pulled me up to a sitting position.

"Efcharisto," I said to them.

"Kalah," they replied.

Then they opened the windows. The air felt nice and wintry. They gave me some bottled water and scurried out, away from the crazy American.

I sat there for a moment and pondered my ridiculous fate. I wondered what the hell was wrong with me. Nothing like this had happened since 1990 when I had ended up in the hospital, paralyzed for more than a month.

With my two legs hanging off the side of the bed, I fell back and slept again. Hours later, I woke up and called Dr. Kountouris's office.

"Stella," I said, "Please tell the doctor that I'm sick and can't move."

Dr. Kountouris called back an hour later and told me to sit tight, as I had obviously contracted an infection. He said he would send someone over with medicine.

The doctor's office was only a block away, but still it took Christo, his assistant, four hours to show up with some pills. I could tell by his eyes he felt badly for me.

Christo didn't speak English very well, but he tried to reach out to me in a language I could understand.

"Play blues, Gary!" he said and gave me the thumbs up.

I nodded weakly and said, *"Efcharisto,* Christo."

When he left, I sat there and cursed Dr. Kountouris and cursed Athens and cursed my doctor back in the States for being right. I realized what Doctor D. had meant when he had warned me that my immune system might be suppressed from the treatment. I guess that meant that I was vulnerable to anything.

Then Theo walked through the door, just like Superman. He picked me up, moved me to the other bed and hooked me up to two bags of IV antibiotics he hung from the closet door.

I asked him what had happened to me.

"Don't know," he said.

I told him he had saved my life. He just laughed.

"That crazy communist," I thought. He always seemed to bring me back to life.

Within an hour, I was up and walking around again. I would need my cane for a few days to walk, but, amazingly, it didn't take long to recover from this setback.

My last night in Athens: I'm lying on a table in Dr. Kountouris's office getting a final dose of immunoglobulin, which had been administered to me along with the chemotherapy.

Dr. D. comes in with Anastasia to give me his parting instructions and farewells.

He warns me of the importance of keeping up my morale, what he calls my "psycho balance."

And he reminds me of the story about the bird.

Once there was a bird that flew to the top of a mountain. He enjoyed his time on top, but he soon wondered what it would be like to fly back down to the world below. He flew effortlessly down the mountain, not realizing what a struggle it would be to fly back up again.

I will need, Dr. D. emphasizes, to fly smoothly and evenly from now on, or it will become more difficult each time to get back to the top.

Though I leave Athens not needing my cane or my wheelchair, it isn't a miracle yet. The effects of the treatment will have to last, and I know now that miracles can take a long time to reveal themselves.

I could not continue the treatment when I returned to the States. The effects from the mitoxantrone did not last.

Dr. Kountouris couldn't locate anyone in the medical community who would help. The treatment I had received in Greece was not prescribed for MS in the United States. No one, of course, wanted to break the rules.

Dr. D. wrote to me and recommended that I take metheltrexate as a supplement until I could continue the mitoxantrone treatment. At the time, however, that was not something I was willing to do. Although metheltrexate is prescribed in the States for treating MS, I was still afraid of the side effects.

I returned home to find my wife wanted a divorce, so the end of my journey was tempered with disappointment and pain. It seems the problems we had faced before my trip to Greece had increased in my absence.

I came to realize, though, that the journey itself had inspired me; memories are powerful antidotes.

I will always remember my taxi ride to the top of Lacavitos, the mountain with the famous Greek Orthodox church on top. I went there to yell my son Jamie's name from the top, having promised I would yell it so loudly that he would hear me all the way from Greece.

As I made my way to the top of that mountain on a bright, clear day, I was full of hope. Below me, I could see the city of Athens stretching its arms toward the sea. Facing home, I envisioned my son asleep in his bed, maybe dreaming of me. I yelled his name, loudly and boldly, the force of the sound containing my hope. I wanted to walk through the door when I returned home and lift my son into the air. I wanted to dance through the kitchen with my wife, ride through the streets of my hometown, my daughter's legs dangling from the handlebars of my bike. When I yelled Jamie's name on top of the mountain, I was hoping to awaken the Gods of fate.

My son has grown in the years since I returned. I was never able to play soccer with him, but I found other ways to be his father. I think he knows that the part of me struggling to get well is the part that loves him most.

During my visit, I was able to set up a recording session at one of the best studios in Athens, where I recorded seven songs with some incredible musicians. I had been in need of something besides the doctor's office, and the musicians I met made me feel at home. The positive and, perhaps, curative power of music is something I have known about for a long time. It is one of the more purely satisfying experiences I had on my journey to Athens.

A few months after leaving Athens, I heard that Theo had suffered a heart attack and was no longer working for Dr. Kountouris. He later moved to northern Greece.

I returned to Greece a few years after my first visit. This time, it was not to find a cure—at least, not a medical cure. I wanted to laugh with Theo again and look into the far distance for the Parthenon, sitting gracefully beyond the dull concrete homes of the city.

I wanted to yell from the mountaintops and remember what had made me whole.

GARY SHANE LAVENSON *was a performing musician in the Boston area in the 1970s and 1980s. He now works as a real estate sales representative and still enjoys writing songs. He lives on a lake in Amesbury, Massachusetts.*

3

RECREATING A LIFE

Kathleen Wilson

In the fall of 1993, I was living in Athens, Greece. I was lured back there by memories of a trip I had taken many years before, when I had produced some of my best artwork. My fascination with the light and colors of Greece remained deeply within me, and I felt a strong need to return.

Greece is the place that helped me find my best expression as a photographer. In Athens, the light seemed to reach into the core of things and reveal the essence of something deeper than surface appearance. This is especially true of the water there.

Water had been my photographic passion for fifteen years, and I found the water in Athens to be the most spectacular, especially in the nearby port of Piraeus.

My life in Athens was a simple one. I was fortunate to live in Plaka, the ancient part of the city surrounding the base of the Acropolis. My apartment was minimal, a mere basement with windows that opened to a dusty, dirty, well-trafficked road.

> MY SPIRIT RUNS DEEP,
> AND WITHIN IT
> ARE ALL OF THE TOOLS
> THAT I NEED TO
> REINVENT MY LIFE.

During the warmest days of August, I would ride with a friend by motorcycle, south toward the tip of Greece. If we were not going to Sounion, where the temple of Poseidon looks out to the sea, we would stop along the highway at a beautiful swimming area known only to the locals. We would hike down through rugged terrain and find a flat spot on the bleached boulders where we could dive directly into the aquamarine water below. These were the loveliest of days, the moments I felt most content in Greece, surrounded and enveloped by her beauty.

Photographing the aqua-blue sea became part of my weekly ritual while living in Greece. I looked for the imagery within the abstract surfaces. I walked from

morning till mid afternoon, seeking out various ports
where the richest visual material lie in wait. Ironically,
water was the very thing that would end my journey in
Greece, forcing me to embark on a new life path.

After spending a year in Athens, I decided to extend
my stay. I began studying the Greek language at a learning institute in the center of Athens. I wanted to become
more fluent, thinking it might help to broaden my day-to-
day experience. My art was flourishing, and my social
group was growing.

Upon completion of a one-month intensive course, I
began taking private language lessons. It's funny how
being in Greece has a way of inspiring grand intellectual
pursuits. I smile now, remembering the struggle and difficulty that I experienced trying to learn the language.
But I was in love with life, in love with being there. I felt
indestructible and confident.

Three to four times a week, I hopped on my motorbike
and sped off to a local gym. One day, late in March, I was
running late and did something that would forever
change my life. Hurrying through the kitchen, I reached
for some water and, seeing that our water bottle was
empty, I did the forbidden. I drank from the tap. That one
little sip of water would be the beginning of the end of
my time in Greece.

The following morning I awoke with severe abdominal cramps, flu-like symptoms and extreme fatigue. My housemate called around and discovered that a virus, or "micro-bit," as the Greeks call it, had entered the water system, and the entire area surrounding us was contaminated. I had ingested this thing, and like everyone else in our area, I was sick as a dog for days with diarrhea, nausea and other symptoms. I noticed, though, after a week in bed, that when everyone else was recovered, I was still experiencing a bit of fatigue.

I resumed my schedule as soon as I could, but with a lot less vigor. Unable to continue the walks, I scheduled a Greek lesson to help me get back into the swing of things. My love for life seemed a little flat, and I hoped that getting my life on track again would bring me around. In the recesses of my mind, however, was a nagging fear, a fear that I worked hard to repress. I feared that the fatigue might be related to a vision loss that I had endured seven years before, when multiple sclerosis had been mentioned as a possibility.

In early April, while traveling via taxi to my Greek lesson, I noticed a slight tingling in my right hand. When during my language lesson I had difficulty writing, I knew then that something was wrong. Believing that this would go away in a few days, I refused to consider a more serious possibility.

The days grew longer and less interesting. I found it more difficult each day to walk the usual paths, so I walked shorter routes and started leaving my camera at home. In the morning, I would walk to my favorite café, as I always had, and wave to my friends, though I started to notice concern reflected in their faces. My right leg had become rather stiff, but I was still walking. I would shrug my shoulders at my friends and smile until they smiled back, reassuring them that I was fine. I convinced myself that my life would not change, and that I would be back to normal in a few days. Determination is one of my stronger characteristics, but this time it actually prevented me from seeking help.

After three falls at home—once in the bathtub, where I nearly hit my head—I decided to telephone my neurologist in the States. My heart was telling me that my life was changing. I knew that making this call was an admission that something was wrong with me that could not be fixed. Failing health was guiding my decisions now, and I did what was necessary.

It is remarkable to me how our greatest strengths can become our greatest weaknesses. I have developed a gift of persuasion that can sometimes work against me. I convinced my neurologist that Valium and rest might take care of the situation, though he strongly recommended that I return home for treatment.

By mid-June, the end of my stay was in sight. I was still walking but with great difficulty. The need to go home had become greater than my denial and desire to remain. With tears in my eyes, I telephoned my dad and told him that it was time for me to return. Something had taken control of my body, something I could not wrestle into submission.

My housemate helped me pack a few things, although not everything, because I planned to return.

A plane ticket from my parents arrived within the week, leaving me only a few days before I would depart this place of beauty. My heart was broken; the defeat was overwhelming and the changes ahead were unthinkable. I tried to see everyone before I left, reassuring them that as soon as I recovered they would see me again. It was a time of deep remorse. I was losing the life I'd made for myself in the charming and chaotic world of Athens.

On the long plane ride home, I felt helpless to do anything except be the person I was at the moment, a person who could barely walk, heading toward an unknown future. If ever I experienced hopelessness, this was the time. I looked forward to seeing my wonderful parents, always so supportive and present, but I also felt failure, failure as a human being not well enough to take on the task of living.

While shopping duty-free at the airport, I bought a Swiss army watch that I had wanted. Just then it was a distraction, but it became a symbol of time for me, a time of great change. It is a badge of courage and a reminder of where my life today took root.

By the time we reached New York, I was beginning to feel pretty tired, but the thought of seeing my dad there helped me get through customs. Dad had been in New York on business and was able to meet me halfway. I felt joy at seeing him, and he looked at me as though I were in tip-top condition. His positive energy flowed through me, and for a short time, I felt that somehow my illness was just a temporary setback. I'd be back together in no time.

The next flight would take me to Oregon via Salt Lake City, where my mom would meet me. I'll never forget the sight of my beautiful mother when I arrived, waiting and smiling for me, even though our plane was six hours late.

If anything is clear to me about those next six months, it is the gift of laughter that I shared with my mom. Every day brought new challenges. I recall sitting in the passenger seat of the car every time we went somewhere, watching the trunk open, and seeing, through the tiny space between the trunk lid and the car, fragments of my mother hoisting the wheelchair into the trunk. Then she would cheerfully get behind the wheel, and off we would go to the next doctor's appointment or errand.

More than once we were faced with the Oregon rain, unable to see twenty feet in front of us, and we would begin to laugh. We would laugh uncontrollably until our sides hurt, grateful to be alive. We laughed at the impossibility of the moment, the absurdity of life's demands. Humor is a necessary part of survival, and laughing dissolved so much of the pain that I felt every day. I believe that humor is a salve for the soul and the spark that ignites healing.

In remembering this time now, I realize that my mom was my primary caretaker. Mom was the person who drove me everywhere, cooked my meals, cleaned my clothes, helped me to brush my teeth, laughed with me, cried with me and even picked me up when I fell. This was a time when I had to let people help me. It was a difficult part of my journey, because I felt so terrible about myself. On the other hand, I think my apathy at this time toward life allowed me to just go with the flow. Mom kept me tethered to the real world, even though I felt quite detached. Her daily coaching had me going through the motions, so that I never let go completely.

I had arrived home in June 1995, and after two months of failed plasma therapy and physical therapy, I was near giving up. One day blended into the next, and I spent most of my time watching TV, sleeping and doing only what was required of me. Even brushing my teeth had become a major task, not to mention bathing, dressing and sitting up. I could do nothing. I was deeply depressed. Even though supportive friends and family surrounded me, I felt isolated. I no longer belonged to this world, and I felt the world didn't belong to me either. This was the lowest point in my life, and I was too tired to do anything about it.

While watching TV near the end of August, a special program came on about the actor Christopher Reeve. It sparked my interest, so I watched intently as the story of his last two months unfolded. The riding accident that had paralyzed him happened in June of that year, and here he was on the television program *20/20,* giving an interview with Barbara Walters, while I lay in bed feeling sorry for myself. I was so impressed with his determination and positive attitude. It helped me to remember that I, too, had some of that in me. In fact, I had a lot of that in me! This was the very moment I began to realize I could make the climb back to life; the map was within my heart.

One of the first things I did after watching that program was to switch neurologists. Within three days, I was taking the traditional IV steroids. Within twenty-four hours, I was feeling the beneficial result. Any change was monumental to me at this time, and slight improvements were all I needed to begin to feel I might rebuild my life. With the process of reinventing begun, I moved ahead with tiny steps, determined I would not accept defeat.

But taking these steps was not easy for me. I could not remember a time in my life before this MS attack when

I questioned my independence or ability to engage. Now every movement was an effort. The fatigue was overwhelming, forcing me to sleep for several hours during the day.

My world gained some focus, slowly. My spirit began to reemerge, and I started to feel conscious and aware. Hopeful there might be more for me than sitting home feeling dependent on everyone else for all of my needs, I began creating a new life for myself.

One day, my mom approached me with a very important question. She asked if anything on the planet could improve the quality of my life. I thought for a moment and without hesitation said, "A computer." For the first time in months, I was feeling a genuine desire to do something. We both got a little excited, and that very afternoon I came home with a brand new Mac Performa.

During that month and into the next, as my strength returned, I began to learn about the computer and I went online to read about MS. There was real information that I could relate to, and I found answers to the many questions swimming in my brain. This machine was more than just a computer to me. It reconnected me to the world, engaging my interest and giving me a sense of belonging. Deeply inspired, I let my heart be my compass.

I could feel myself entering a phase full of possibility. The very first time I visited a chat room, I knew that this format was critical for those of us who were shut off from the world. I was exhilarated and kept searching other chat rooms until I found one for people with disabilities.

This was a joyous time. The world came to me via the computer, sparking my need to create. I had forgotten my art, having left it in Athens with the rest of my old life. I could see there was no going back. I now took another step toward reinventing and reassembling my shattered life, applying my creativity with all my heart and soul.

When my parents and I moved back to our winter home in Sarasota, I continued rebuilding the life that had been thrown into chaos just four months earlier. I had little desire to return to the past, though friends in Greece still awaited my return. I accepted that I would have to disappoint them in order to move forward.

By early December, I located a local university that offered a master's degree in mental health counseling. The wonderful thing about this program was that I could begin coursework online and attend classes when I was strong enough to do so. With one master's degree already completed, I was admitted to the counseling program in February 1996 and began courses that spring. This was exactly the distraction and challenge I needed to get going. Fortunately, my computer would help me not only with the online course work, but also to write the many papers that would be required over the next two years.

It felt so good to be involved in the real world again. I was happy to take the place of an equal among others. The people I met along the way looked at me with a great deal of respect and offered only positive encouragement. My instructors were very accommodating as well, and agreed to let me take oral exams because of my difficulty in writing.

In July, I decided to create my own MS chat room online. I had been involved with a chat room for people with disabilities, but I wanted to create a resource on the Internet for MS alone, one that would offer information and support about the disease in a positive and helpful way. The chat room I had been participating in was a bit depressing and unorganized. People with every ailment under the sun congregated there, making it difficult to find a real sense of belonging or to gather helpful information about any one illness. I obtained some training on the technical aspects of running an online chat and began what would eventually grow into MSWorld, Inc.

MSWorld, Inc. (*www.msworld.org*) is now a nonprofit organization providing comprehensive support and information via the Internet to people with multiple sclerosis. The site has grown to include daily chat, e-mail groups, message boards, a resource library, research articles, book reviews, guest speakers and an online magazine. Thousands of people around the world have accessed MSWorld seeking support, reliable information and assistance in making informed health decisions. MSWorld also provides strategies for coping with the difficulties of living with a chronic illness.

This is where my inner landscape finds expression these days. From the very first chat, the growth of MSWorld has been steady and constant. Within two months, I assembled a staff of six from all over the world, each bringing unique talents to help create a solid and truly helpful organization.

MS has taught me that life isn't so much about recovery as it is about self-discovery. It has opened within me other avenues for growth. My spirit runs deep, and within it are all the tools I need to reinvent my life. When we are willing to reinvent ourselves, we impact those around us. When we change for the better and share what we have learned, we help others to adopt better ways of living as well. In this way, I have been able to contribute to the world beyond myself.

When I left behind the blue-green seas of Athens, having put away my camera and my dreams, the future seemed like a vast and empty canvas. I see now that the emptiness was merely an invitation to create, and this I have done. Our slogan at MSWorld sums it up: "Wellness is a state of mind."

KATHLEEN WILSON *has been making photographic pictures for over twenty years. With several gallery shows to her credit, she now pursues her visionary art in Sarasota, Florida. Kathleen's pictures are exhibited in a gallery that also serves as the office for MSWorld, Inc., the Web site she created for people with multiple sclerosis. The proceeds from her gallery sales are donated to MSWorld. Some of her work can be seen at the online magazine* LivingMS *(www.msworld.org).*

4 STAGES

Nina Gendell

SHOCK AND DENIAL

Yesterday my baby turned four-and-one-half months old. He's soft and clean-smelling, all bright eyes and velvety smiles. His image is a sharp contrast to the man sitting across from me naming possibilities. A lesion on the optic nerve. A brain tumor pressing on the optic nerve. Multiple sclerosis.

The man is unkempt. The pockets of his trousers are frayed at the binding. His hair is thick, stiff and dark with oil. He looks like he should be selling insurance or managing freight shipments from a dusty and cluttered office. Instead he is dispensing a life-altering medical diagnosis from a sunny tower with a picturesque view. And he has no smiles for me.

For some reason my jaw falls at the mention of multiple sclerosis. I have to remind myself to breathe. Later I wonder why. A lesion on the optic nerve or a brain tumor is just as bad. Perhaps I know intuitively that this is what is wrong with me. He seems to notice that I twitch and goes on to tell me in a cold monotone that MS does not interfere with the daily activities of many people, that he's not just "gilding the lily." I wonder what that cliché means. I've heard it a thousand times before, but never bothered to find out what it means. It is a strange phrase. What would be the point of putting a thin layer of gold on a lily?

> LEARNING TO MANAGE AND LIVE WITH MS CAN BE TRICKY, BUT PARENTHOOD IS A MUCH MORE DEFINING AND POWERFUL ROLE.

I shut off and concentrate on the bright image of my perfect little boy sitting with his dad in the small, airless waiting room. I imagine the feel of his warm, squirming body on my lap. He will be full of smiles and absolute, adoring love for me when I walk out the door that is separating us—no matter how bad the news. His shiny eyes will search my face and lock with my eyes, and a buttery grin will spread across his face, tempting me to melt. But I will concentrate on steeling myself, not allowing for the possibility that I may not be physically capable of giving him the happy childhood I've planned.

The doctor is droning on about an MRI: a brain scan more accurate than the CT scan I'd had a few days ago. He wants me to have one urgently. If I go to a private clinic, I can have one immediately, but it will cost $500 and is not refundable through Medicare. If I go to a public hospital, it will be free, but I will have to wait two to three weeks. My friend Pippa had to wait months to get on the free list at a public hospital—and she had a brain tumor. It's urgent, he stresses. Nobody has ever ordered a test urgently on my behalf before. If it's likely to be MS and MS won't interfere with my daily activities, why do I need an MRI urgently? I press my "off" button, tell him I'll wait for a booking at a public hospital and dash out to my baby as soon as I can without seeming rude. Afterward, I wonder why I cared about my manners when he didn't have enough regard for his patients to wash his hair.

Later, my husband is filled with questions, but I don't know the answers. I'd switched off and floated through the man's droning, clutching my baby in my mind's eye, rather than thinking about the lesions in my brain. I am on automatic, waiting to hear from Prince of Wales

Hospital about a date for my "urgent" MRI. I do the same things I did yesterday—shovel orange purée into my baby's mouth, load the dishwasher, cook, eat, watch television. Waiting is stressful. I want a diagnosis so I can begin to deal with whatever I've got.

Anger

10 June 1998
Dr. Con Maxwell
Sydney Eye Hospital
Macquarie Street
SYDNEY 2000

Dear Dr. Maxwell:

I am writing in the hope that you will be interested in some feedback from an emergency patient.

I was referred to the emergency room at the Sydney Eye Hospital on 16 April by my general practitioner. At the time, I was blind in one eye. I was very impressed by how quickly and efficiently I was looked after. I found you to be professional and courteous; however, I wish you had been straight with me about your suspicions.

In retrospect, it is clear from the questions you asked that you suspected multiple sclerosis from the outset. Instead of discussing health care options with me, you made an appointment and referred me directly to Dr. Milton Dander, whom you described as an ophthoneurologist. At the time, I was overwhelmed by my mysterious blindness, knowing that healthy thirty-seven-year-old women don't go blind in one eye for no reason. I was also preoccupied with my baby, who was forced to spend a long day cooped up in his carriage. I assumed that Dr. Dander was some sort of "super" specialist and that you had good reasons for referring me to him. I didn't think to question you at the time, because you acted as if you had no idea what was wrong with me.

I will assume that you have never met Dr. Dander. If you had, you would know that he practices poor hygiene, appalling grooming and is completely lacking in bedside manner. If you have met him, shame on you for referring me. He led me to believe that I was seriously ill with either MS or a brain tumor and sent me away in a tailspin, worried that I wouldn't be able to look after my gorgeous child as he grew up. He impressed me with the urgency of getting an MRI as soon as possible.

To make a long story short, he wasn't able to get me onto the MRI free list for three months. I rang my general practitioner, got a referral to the MS clinic in Sydney (a much easier location to get to from home than Bondi Junction) and was consulted by a professor who explained the disease to me in a sensitive and personable fashion. He was able to schedule an MRI two days later (at a private clinic, paid for by the MS Society). He assured me that I have a mild case and advised me to get on with my life. My diagnosis was confirmed within a week.

The point of all of this is that if you had discussed your suspicions with me as a doctor to an adult, I would have had the option of taking control of my own health care from the start and would have been spared a good deal of unnecessary stress and emotional upset. I can appreciate that as a registrar and ophthalmologist you may not have been keen to offer a neurological diagnosis, but you could have discussed your suspicions with me. Why didn't you suggest optic neuritis as a possible explanation for my blindness, explain that it is a neurological disorder and that it was why you were referring me to a neurologist? I just can't help wondering if you would have been so furtive with a thirty-seven-year-old male patient presenting with the same symptoms.

At any rate, I thank you for your expert care on the day and for recognizing my symptoms as neurological, even though you didn't share that information with me. I hope you can appreciate my feedback.

Sincerely,
Nina Gendell

SADNESS

I let the baby sleep late on a Friday afternoon. Usually, I wake him by 4:00, so that he is ready to go to bed at 7:00 and I can enjoy a quiet evening. I look at the clock. It is 4:26. I switch on the TV so I don't miss the beginning of *The Bold and the Beautiful.* I have been following the damn show for months and always miss the opening titles when I switch on at 4:30.

I catch the end of a children's drama series. It must only be screened on Fridays. At home with a baby, I thought I knew the daytime television schedule by heart. *Totally Wild* is on every other day. As the credits scroll, I notice it is made by a production company my friend Paul worked for. I scan the screen for his name, but hardly expect the final credit, a dedication to his memory. I am surprised by the sob that pounds the back of my throat and the tears rolling down my cheeks. Tears that didn't escape at his funeral. Not even when his teenage niece got up in front of the recycled timber coffin, covered with Australian wildflowers, and sang a bluesy solo version of *Amazing Grace.*

As the tears roll, I think about Paul crashing to his death. Going out in a blaze of glory. The moment of impact, skidding across the road, head smashing pavement through his helmet, skin tearing from flesh through shredded clothing. I wonder if he ever had the time to think "Oh shoot!" If he was aware of the oncoming loss of consciousness. If there was enough time for pain.

I imagine Paul would have preferred to lose control in the drama of a motorbike crash, rather than in the insipid silence of a hospital bed. I'd visited him in the hospital several times over the years. Wan, pale, immobile, his blood like water, trying to keep the mysterious clots from journeying to his brain.

That Friday afternoon, as the tears roll down my cheeks, I suddenly realize how much I miss Paul. I am sad that he died before he met my baby. And I grieve, because I am sick like he was. I have to live with the time bomb of MS for the rest of my life, never knowing if and when it might detonate, leaving me with a brain that can still think and rationalize, a sergeant that can't relay commands to private functions—bladder, bowel, limbs. An otherwise healthy body that will cease to operate. Bit by bit.

I grieve, because in a short time, I have lost a friend and I have lost my health.

BARGAINING

I try to read *You Can Heal Your Life* by Louise Hay. Both Pippa and Margaret recommend it. Though I trust their judgment, I reserve it at the library rather than rushing out to buy it as I usually would. I always find self-help books hard to stomach, so I skip to the last chapter to read Hay's own story. She tells of a life of abuse, lost love and then cancer. A "mental pattern" ("deep resentment" in her case) created illness, and a change in thinking cured it. The story leaves me sure that I created my multiple sclerosis with negative thought and I have the power to make it go away with positive thought, just as she did. My psychiatrist tells me this is dangerous psychology. She says I run the risk of blaming myself for being ill. And for a while, I do blame myself.

I am shattered. I must have created MS, because I am no good at positive thinking. Defeated and depressed, I return the book to the library, glad I didn't buy it. I don't want it sitting around my house, staring at me from a shelf, a constant reminder of how weak I am, how stupid I've been to get myself into something I can't easily get out of.

It baffles me. The disease has struck at a time when I've finally achieved a degree of contentment—happy marriage, delightful baby, reasonable finances. But while I've always had a job, I've never had a career. My negative thoughts all tend to merge and disperse from there. MS could easily be the perfect reason for me to give up trying to achieve the thing that is missing in my life.

For most of my adult life, I have been mired in anxiety when it comes to employment. I have never made the right decision when facing a crossroad in my working life. I do the safe thing: find something I do well and do it for so long that neither I nor my employer can see me doing anything different.

I start having conversations with my disease. I confess that when I meet someone new, I always avoid the question "So, what do you do for a living?" I have always bemoaned, "I don't know what I want to be when I grow up." I tried law school but found that the law has nothing to do with justice. Disillusioned, I dropped out and have been groping for something else ever since. Now I am precariously close to forty and still don't know "what I want to be."

I want to blame someone. I know that if I had a satisfying career, I could think positive thoughts all the time and make MS go away. For a while I blame my parents for making me afraid of taking risks in my working life. My father always wanted to strike out on his own and do freelance work, but my mother always wanted him to play it safe and work for a boss, bring home a regular wage—like her father did. As a child, I remember my parents fighting about it at night. I remember the terrifying thunder of "Go back to bed!" when I'd get up to investigate. But blaming them leaves me squelching through a deep swamp of negative thoughts.

My disease emerges from the morass in the form of a large, dark persona. He holds it over my head that I've never found a way to get paid for being the creative person I know I am. I try to explain to him that nothing has ever felt right. I have been waiting, secretly hoping that some day I would be in the right place at the right time. Someone would see my talent, and the perfect job would fall into my lap. I'd go from strength to strength, enjoy getting up to go to work each day, make lots of money and never look back. It's not really my fault that it has never happened, I whine. And I thrash myself in the presence of multiple sclerosis. He knows I am weak.

I plead with my disease to go easy on me, because I have become so subsumed by administrative duties— forms, filing, lists, rosters—that I can feel my intelligence and imagination dripping out like a slow leak in an oil tank, leaving me feeling rusted and dry. I have lost the confidence to pursue anything creative. I stroke my disease, trying to keep him calm.

He stares at me coldly. I decide to return to work rather than stay at home indefinitely with my baby. MS could easily become another excuse in my growing list of excuses to give up on pursuing a career. I whisper gently to my disease and promise to develop my creative side. He looks cynical—but doesn't advance as I pull myself from the swamp.

I consider Louise Hay's list of metaphysical causes of illness. According to her, MS is caused by "mental hardness" (what does that mean?), "hard-heartedness" (not me!), "iron will" (maybe), "inflexibility" (sometimes), "fear" (I must confess). I shove Louise Hay into a cupboard in the back of my mind and snap the door shut. Multiple sclerosis howls in the distance.

ACCEPTANCE

Looking at my positive pregnancy test, I cried. I wanted a baby badly, but I was filled with a sense of foreboding. I was sure something would go wrong. I couldn't believe it when he was born without a crossed eye or a mark on his rabbit-soft skin.

While childbirth doesn't cause MS, it is common for an attack to occur in the months following birth. Because of the timing, the diagnosis of MS will always be inextricably linked in my mind to the birth of my baby. Yet it never occurred to me that the anxiety I felt when staring at that pregnancy test was misdirected, meant for me. Wasn't it enough that I had four days of false labor and no sleep followed by an emergency cesarean? Hadn't I paid my dues? What did I do to deserve such a kick with the proverbial steel-tipped boot while I was down?

I make a mental list of all the grief I have suffered in my life:

1. Father abandoned family when I was twelve.
2. Brother diagnosed with reactive schizophrenia shortly after my father left.

3. Mother forced to raise me and my brothers on public assistance.
4. Broken heart once when I was eighteen and even worse when I was twenty-one.

I don't need to make a complete and thorough list to know that I have endured my fair share. Multiple sclerosis is simply one more to add to the list. Something else I'll get through.

When I was diagnosed, Pippa was the first person I told. She's been sick, and she knew what I was going through. She said getting sick was the best thing that ever happened to her, because she'd learned how to filter out the unimportant things, enjoy life, make every day count. I'm not so good at being positive and am not sure how to make every day of relative health count.

Going to MS support group meetings helps. I learn several points of interest:

1. It is unwise to tell everyone, especially at work, because they can make assumptions about whether you are still capable of doing your job.
2. Employers can force sick employees out of work before they are ready to go.
3. People can be cruel without intending to be. Friends don't know how to deal with you as a sick person when they have always known you as a well person.

4. A person in a wheelchair or someone who is incontinent can still have a great sense of humor and a meaningful life.

I am not quite so afraid any more.

I meet a man at one of these meetings. He's furious that his disease has had the audacity to invade his once super-fit body. He was diagnosed two-and-a-half years ago, and talks about going through eighteen months of extreme anger. He talks about blocking out family and friends, locking his door, and retreating to his computer. He talks about diving into bed and screaming his lungs out into his pillow. I wonder how he perceives his attitude now, if not angry. He asks repeatedly how I cope with different things, and I tell him again and again that I am lucky to have my baby to focus on. I am glad that I am not as angry as he is.

I make a list of my current symptoms:

1. Loss of some motor control
2. Pins and needles and a tremor in my left hand
3. Pins and needles in my feet
4. Frequent urination, especially at night
5. Bowel urgency
6. Clumsiness
7. Fatigue
8. Insomnia
9. Heat sensitivity
10. Fear

Things could be a lot worse. Steroids seem to have restored my vision. I no longer go blind in my right eye every time I am too warm. I occasionally get frustrated with my left hand, but have learned to hide its uselessness. I am grateful that my right hand is unaffected. I can still do most things, like type and do up buttons, though it takes more concentration now. I laugh at myself and apologize when I stumble in front of other people, even though I neither think it is funny nor feel sorry. Meditation and yoga help the fatigue and insomnia. I have learned to rest regularly without feeling guilty and to save steps. (Energy is like money in the bank, you have to save it in order to spend it, according to the MS Society's occupational therapist.) I am not in any pain. My baby is a happy child, amused by the games I invent for him, even when I don't move much while we play.

I used to wonder which I would have chosen if I could have seen into the future—a life of relative health and no baby, or multiple sclerosis with a baby. Who knows if MS would have ever attacked if I hadn't given birth?

I make a list of the things I love about my son:

1. The beautiful contours of his perfect little body
2. The curve of his eyelashes
3. The way he giggles when I wipe the poop from his wrinkly scrotum
4. His smile, especially when he purses his lips and looks just like me when I was a little girl

5. His expressive vocabulary— "ningan ningan" when he is complaining, "tigga tigga" when he is up to mischief and "gudga gudga" when he is pleased
6. The rounded pads on the bottom of each of his big toes that haven't flattened, because he isn't walking yet

I know now that even if I'd been given the choice, I would have chosen the magical experience of motherhood. I decide that I will not be defined by my illness. Learning to manage and live with MS can be tricky, but parenthood is a much more defining and powerful role. My child embraces new experiences and approaches each day with delight. My life is enriched and constantly moving forward when viewing the world through his eyes.

NINA GENDELL *has been living in Sydney, Australia, for the past twelve years, although she is a native New Yorker. Amid the chaos of home renovating, chasing after a toddler and working part-time, she escapes to the cinema as often as possible, reads avidly, enjoys cooking, swimming, yoga, and slouching in front of the TV, and has traveled extensively throughout Europe, Asia, America, and Australia. Nina is married and has two children.*

5 FAMILY

Dave Perez

I was twenty-seven years old when I realized that the plans we make for our lives are sometimes secondary to circumstance. I was then a single father, alone and raising three children.

If you had told me years before that I would be the center of my children's universe, I might not have believed you. But life is unpredictable. I can still remember a time when I had never heard of multiple sclerosis.

❖ ❖ ❖ ❖

In June of 1986, I was a newlywed with a son. I was on top of the world and moving right along through the ranks of the Navy, training at an engineering school near Chicago. After so many dead-end jobs, I was finally directing my life in a fulfilling way.

Just a few months later, while working the midnight to 4:00 A.M. watch, I awoke to find that my left eye wouldn't clear up from its "sleep mode." As night turned into day, I became a bit concerned—though not enough to go to the doctor's office. I am one of those people who wait until their arm falls off before seeking medical attention.

> I GUESS YOU CAN SAY I AM ON A MISSION TO BE THE BEST "ME" I CAN BE. I NOW FOCUS ON WHAT I CAN DO AND TAKE IT FROM THERE.

As the days passed, my eye became a little worse; and then the trouble began with my left leg, which felt as if it had fallen asleep and wouldn't wake up. Climbing the ladder at the training facility on the base was becoming very difficult.

I wasn't yet at sea, but I expected to be shipping out in another month to Long Beach, California. That's all the more reason I was hoping this "pinched nerve" would pass. I had been through too much training and had worked too hard, to let this stumbling and vision problem slow the progress of my career.

My stubbornness in seeking medical attention ended when, two weeks later, I became totally blind in one eye. I went to the eye clinic on the base where, despite my condition, I was treated terribly. They actually accused me of bluffing so that I could find a way out of the Navy; when the doctor looked into my eye, he didn't see anything obviously wrong.

When the problem with my eye refused to disappear, I reluctantly made my way to the clinic again. Before whisking me off to the main hospital to see a specialist, the corpsman at the clinic told me that the staff members who had previously examined me had been "talked to" by their superiors for the poor way they had treated me. Finally, a specialist at the hospital found a problem with my optic nerve and I was sent to a neurologist off base.

Like many people who are diagnosed with multiple sclerosis, the day that I first heard those words is forever etched in my memory—February 7, 1987. Each year, February 7 rolls around like some kind of morbid anniversary.

After examining me, the neurologist handed me my medical records and suggested that I go back to my military doctor to discuss my diagnosis. Evidently, she wanted me to be told by "one of my own."

When the military doctor explained to me that I had

multiple sclerosis, he added that he didn't know the first thing about it. After allowing me time to overcome the initial shock, he admitted me immediately to the hospital.

I struggled to keep calm as I drove home to pack my things, but I found myself crying anyway. As I walked in the door, my wife could tell by the look on my face that something was terribly wrong. That's when I finally broke down.

My MS progressed very quickly. Looking back, I think trying to keep up with my Navy buddies and all of our activities might have made it worse. Our platoon leader had a black belt in karate, and he was in charge of our physical training. The members of my platoon and I were on a mission to run as many laps as he did, and then go an extra mile. It didn't matter which exercises we were doing; we always had to have one up on the platoon leader. This wasn't a very practical approach to managing MS, but I hadn't yet learned how to deal with the disease.

After enduring several more attacks, I was sent to Walter Reed Medical Center in Washington, D.C. I spent a month there, isolated from my friends and family—the very people whose support I needed.

Despite the diligent medical attention, there was to be no reprieve. The end of my naval career was in sight. I continued having one attack after another until, suddenly, everything stopped working. First, I lost the use of my legs, and then my arms. I couldn't walk, feed myself or even brush my teeth. People took turns shaving me. It was very hard for me to accept their help. I felt guilty because they were taking time away from their own lives to help me. I found myself thanking them endlessly.

Just as I was getting used to being unable to operate the remote control for the TV, the MS started to affect my breathing. I was admitted to the hospital again, where the doctors told my family that, most likely, I had only a few months to live. One evening, as my family gathered in the hallway outside my room, my doctor approached and asked them to join him in the lounge. He warned them of my dire situation, so when everybody came to say good night, I had the distinct feeling they were paying their last respects to me, although I didn't know why. Their faces were serious, gloomy and sad. It's a good thing I wasn't aware of the doctor's prediction at the time. I've learned that you can't underestimate the power of hope.

Although I wasn't aware of it, the people who loved me were afraid that I would die. I had to stop in mid sentence to take a few short breaths before I could finish speaking my thoughts. It occurred to me that breathing was essential to life, and I, too, began to fear the worst. But after heavy doses of steroids, and with the support of my family, my MS went into remission and I came around again.

During this difficult time, I learned that my wife was expecting our second child. At first I panicked. I didn't know much about multiple sclerosis, and I worried about what effects the disease or the steroids could have on our unborn child. My wife's doctor suggested we have an amniocentesis performed to detect any birth defects; but after some thought and discussion, we decided to go through with the birth without intervention.

After I was discharged from the Navy, there was a lapse before we received any kind of monetary aid. Disability payments from Social Security hadn't started yet, and even when they did, there wasn't enough for us to afford our own place. My mother and stepfather graciously opened their doors to us until my Veteran's Disability kicked in. Two months later, after moving into their home, we were blessed with a beautiful daughter we named Heather. It would only be a matter of months until we could afford a place of our own.

The days before our second child was born were very difficult: I had to crawl through our apartment to get from one room to another. My oldest child, Nick, four years old at the time, always asked if I needed his help and was always willing to do whatever I asked of him. When we went to the store, he would proudly push his daddy's wheelchair or open doors while someone else pushed. He felt most proud at the mall, where we spent some of our more memorable times. I had a T-shirt made up especially for our treks there, which said, "I have MS. MS doesn't have me."

I remember one day an older woman approached us to tell us she admired my shirt. She thought it was wonderful

that I had such an upbeat attitude. As for me, I couldn't
see any way of dealing with this terrible and unpredictable disease other than with positive thinking and a
sense of humor. People often came up to my son and told
him how great he was for helping his dad. I believe those
experiences helped him to see other disabled people as
"normal." I think my children are more sensitive to other
people's needs because of what they live with every day.

When I was growing up, it was considered rude to look
at or approach people who were different from me. But
my children, growing up in a house with a disabled person, came to realize that people with disabilities are still
"normal," even if they tire easily or can't walk. I am very
grateful for that. Not everyone has developed that kind of
sensitivity.

When I went through the process of being honorably
discharged from the Navy, I saw just how insensitive the
world can be; it was a terrible experience. My discharge
papers are a reminder of the poor condition I was in at the
time: The signature does not look anything at all like mine.
I had to hold the pen in my mouth to assist my hand in
signing the endless pile of paperwork. Yet I was treated
very badly, as if I were worthless, wasting everyone's time
with my paperwork. I was using a manual wheelchair and
a friend was pushing me around the base, where it seemed

we had to go to every building for a signature. Each building had stairs, of course, but no ramps for the disabled. Why would they make their buildings accessible? People in the military are healthy enough to climb a few stairs! I especially remember one building in particular, where we had to go up eight flights of stairs. There was an elevator at the rear of the building, but I was told I couldn't use it because it was for freight—not for people.

That was a very long day, during which I encountered two types of people: the ones who looked down on me as if I had no business being in their presence, and those whose compassionate hearts shared words with me that I still remember. The latter were those who wished me the best and offered my friend a hand in pulling me up stairs. The others simply told me to get out of their way because they had somewhere important to go and my wheelchair was blocking their path.

My dreams of having a career in the Navy had come to an end, even though I had carefully mapped out my future: an illustrious career with the military, perhaps leading to a job with the power industry somewhere down the road. Learning to let go of those dreams was difficult. Even now, when I come across news about a power plant that's being designed, my heart sinks and I reminisce about what might have been.

Within a year of my daughter's birth, my wife became pregnant again with our third child, a son we named Matthew. I had worried that having children might be an added hardship to an already difficult situation, but it turned out that the birth of our children was an incredible blessing—just what the doctor ordered. The world no longer revolved around me. I had new and wonderful experiences to deal with—like first words, first steps, potty training. I loved it all. I cherished every moment with the children and still do.

When my wife and I later agreed to a divorce, there was no problem in deciding where the kids should live. We both knew, under the circumstances, that I was in a much better position to raise our children. It was true that I had an unpredictable disease, but the love I had for my children seemed a powerful defense, one that could form a wall around us and help us through the difficult days. Because I was no longer working, I'd be there in the morning to get them up for school and in the afternoon when they returned.

In some ways, I was terrified at the thought of being on my own. I would be solely responsible for three other human beings. What if I had an attack? Who would take care of the kids?

When I began dating again, I think I was subconsciously holding tryouts for a replacement wife. I hadn't developed the confidence I needed to raise my children alone. A few women auditioned for the part, but in the end, I realized that I was doing just fine on my own.

I have always put my children before anything else in my life. They are terrific kids, really—the best. Sometimes when we go somewhere, someone will compliment them on the way they behave and I can't help but beam with pride, as only a parent can do. They've turned out to be very well-mannered children, polite to adults and sensitive to other people's needs. They've grown up with their daddy having MS, and it's given them strong character when it comes to living their own lives.

I can't help, though, feeling a little guilty when I'm unable to participate in certain activities with them. It's hard to watch them ride away on their bikes without me; I want so badly to go. But we've learned to enjoy the things we can do together—like urban hikes. It's not exactly mountainous terrain, but we enjoy strolling through the city together, me in my wheelchair, the kids walking alongside.

We've had to change the way we play a few of our favorite backyard games. With football, I play quarterback—and I stay in one place while everyone else runs around. Then I half run, half stumble a few steps, and lunge toward them. It's the same story with baseball or basketball: I play the most stationary position and try to catch or tag the kids when they get too close.

There are a few activities I just don't get involved in anymore. We have a pool in the backyard, and I like to float around on my air mattress and look up at the clouds. But being in the pool with the kids and their neighborhood friends is a different matter! When I see them heading toward me with their bathing suits on, it's time for me to get out, though they always manage to talk me into staying in for a short time. When I retire to the air conditioning, I look outside to see what madness I'm missing in the pool.

One of my concerns since my diagnosis is how my children will deal with their father not working. I remember when I was young, I used to brag that my dad made railroad track. What were my kids going to brag about? In the society we live in, it seems the first question we are asked when we meet someone is "What do you do for a living?" That's the one question I dread now when meeting someone new. It's also an obstacle when dating. When do I bring up MS? How do I tell them that bike riding is out? There are some wonderful people in the world who don't care if you can't run a marathon—people who accept you for being you. But, sometimes, it feels as if I have to justify my not working, because I look fine and there are no visible clues about why I cannot work. "Looking well" is a problem a lot of people with MS have to deal with every day.

I have gone through many stages while dealing with multiple sclerosis, and I'm sure that they are fairly common: First, I felt fear. I was scared for my future—fearful of how I would manage to provide financially for my family. I was also afraid of what the MS was going to do to me!

Then I got mad. I was mad at the world, mad at God and mad at myself for maybe having done something that caused me to have the disease. When the feelings of anger passed, I began to pity myself. I would cry like a baby in my room, in the shower, any place where no one could see me. Luckily, that part didn't last as long as the other stages I went through. I will say, though, I believe it's therapeutic to feel a little self-pity occasionally—as long as you don't rain on anyone else's parade.

The fourth stage of dealing with my disease was acceptance. I had to learn to accept what I could and could not do. Eventually I learned to say no. (That one took a while!) I had a hard time accepting that I couldn't help my brothers or my friends when they were looking for men to dig a hole or work on other physical tasks. Hard labor is what I grew up with, and it was a big part of my life. I had always been the one who was willing to climb a tree or crawl under a house to jack up a foundation. Now I had to learn how to do things with brain-power instead of elbow grease.

Although my life has changed, I have managed to continue some of my hobbies. I have always loved working on cars. I have one in my garage that I call "my baby." I pulled out the engine and transmission and rebuilt them both. It only took three years! With MS, you learn to do things when you have the time and energy.

I still do as much as I can around the house. On a given day, you might find me climbing on my roof to tar a leak—or you might find me stuck on the roof, because I spent all my energy getting up there. I always laugh when I find myself in these situations, and it happens more times than I'd like to admit. After living with this disease for more than thirteen years, I know my limits, but I am still learning the hard way when it comes to doing physical activities.

I am a leader for my son's Cub Scout pack. During our first time hiking together, no one knew which way to go or how long the trail was. We walked and walked until I decided to tell one of the other leaders that I had to stop. We had reached my limit. I knew, based on the distance we'd walked, that I could make it back to the starting point if I had plenty of rest stops along the way. So we turned around. Luckily, another parent was driving, and I was able to crawl into the car and relax on the long drive home. We've taken the same hike every year now for four years, but always this condensed version: stopping at that halfway point to have lunch and then turning around afterward to hike back to the car.

I am grateful that I have a strong support structure in my life. Most of my family members now recognize my limits. I'm in a golf league with my brother. He drives the cart and tries to get as close to the ball as possible to save me from walking those few extra steps. I have never really told him how much that means to me, but I have a feeling that he knows what I mean when I tell him "Thanks for driving." He's also very protective of me when someone makes a comment on my awkward swing, or the strange way that I walk.

My kids are getting older now, their ages ranging from ten to sixteen. A little over two years ago, I felt they were ready to handle being on their own after school for a few hours. So I called the Chicago-Greater Illinois Chapter of the National Multiple Sclerosis Society (NMSS), and inquired about being a peer counselor. I've been there more than two years now, and I find it very rewarding. I commute from my house to downtown Chicago twice a week. It feels completely natural to talk to people on the phone about MS. I have personally experienced a full range of MS symptoms, and this experience comes in handy when callers ask about a tingling in their arms or legs, or when they explain that they cannot feed themselves. Knowing I have made a difference in someone else's life satisfies me tremendously.

My life has taken a new direction. Once, I had my sights set on a naval career, but now I am focused and determined to help others deal with this disease. I guess you can say I am on a mission to be the best "me" I can be. I now focus on what I can do and take it from there.

In 1990, I received the Father of the Year Award from my NMSS chapter. I was nominated by a member of my local support group. I was very excited to have won the award, although I sincerely believe that the real honor comes from being a father. When the alarm clock rings in the morning, I no longer reach for my Navy dress blues. Instead, I make pancakes, I look for book bags and sneakers, and I rush to get the kids on the bus before it rounds the corner.

My life is quite different from what I had imagined as a young man. But the cards were dealt, and after many discards, I think I have emerged with a winning hand.

DAVE PEREZ *was selected as "Father of the Year" for the Chicago Greater Illinois Chapter of the National MS Society in 1990, and was nominated again in 1999. He is actively involved in the Illinois chapter as a peer support counselor. He recently parachuted from a plane to raise money for MS. He enjoys golfing and spending time with his children. Dave's e-mail address is* ICYOU88@aol.com.

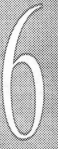

STAYING THE COURSE

Diane Earhart

I was bitten by the flying bug when I was twelve years old. My father had just earned his pilot's license, and on his first flight, he took the family up in a Cessna into the skies over Wisconsin.

It was a life-defining moment for me. Two minutes before the flight, I had no plans for my future; two minutes after the flight, it seemed my entire life was mapped out before me. I knew that I wanted to be a pilot and live my life in the air.

Flying became a part of our lives. Over the next few years, our family flew whenever we could. We'd fly to northern Wisconsin for a picnic, or to visit friends and relatives all over the country. My father promised me that when the time came I, too, could get my license.

To me, flying is sheer joy and freedom in its purest form. Leaving the ground, it feels as if your soul is soaring without the weight of your body. There's the satisfying roar of the engine as the throttle is pushed forward to produce full power for takeoff. The moment the wheels leave the pavement and you know you're actually flying—well, it's indescribable. When you're in the air, there is so little sensation of actual movement that, sometimes, you can't tell if you're moving at all. Sometimes you'll see a layer of cloud rushing by and you are reminded, once again, that you are racing through the sky. The love of flying is a special feeling that only another pilot can truly appreciate.

AFTER I WAS DIAGNOSED, MY EXPERIENCES IN NONCONFORMITY WOULD SERVE ME WELL.

I made my first solo flight on my sixteenth birthday. When I turned seventeen, I passed the check-ride to obtain my private pilot's license.

When pilots record each flight in a logbook to keep

track of aircraft type and hours flown, it actually becomes a diary of memories. Some flights are more memorable than others. I remember one Saturday morning in particular: I got up before the birds to fly over the Wisconsin Dells Balloon Festival before the predawn launch. The hot-air balloons were laid out flat across the ground in every imaginable color. Slowly, the balloons were inflated one by one, as if some invisible giant were lending its breath to a child's birthday party. Fully inflated, the balloons ascended into the sky to join me in the clouds. It was a magical moment.

I happened to be in Washington, D.C., visiting relatives with a friend when the nation's air traffic controllers went on strike. We watched on television as President Ronald Reagan fired every striking controller. My main concern was getting back to Wisconsin; but my friend Chris implored me to consider becoming an air traffic controller myself. "Why don't you apply?" he asked.

Why not, indeed?

I had missed the deadline for the first wave of new hires, but I took the pre-employment exam in November. My score was satisfactory, but not outstanding. I kept in contact with the Federal Aviation Administration, and eventually, was offered a job at the East St. Louis tower in Illinois. I looked up the location in my Rand-McNally atlas and saw that East St. Louis was just across the Mississippi River from St. Louis, Missouri. Well, of course!

I was given a class date, and in June 1982, I packed up my Oldsmobile and hit the road for the FAA Academy in Oklahoma City. In that first year after the strike, the academy was pumping 300 new hires through every five weeks.

From the very first day, the new students had to deal with negative reinforcement. We were told early and often, "Look to your left, look to your right. At the end of this training period, one of you won't be here."

The last day of training, we took a final test. My final score was 73. I'd passed!

Air traffic controlling is not a job for everyone; but for me, it's perfect. I love the spatial orientation of the aerial ballet, fitting the various kinds and speeds of aircraft together. I love seeing all types of flying machines: from vintage tail draggers to the newest three-engine corporate jets, to blimps and large military airplanes old and new. A friend who is a nurse once told me, "I wouldn't be an air traffic controller for all the money in the world!" I say, there's not enough money in the world to make me be a nurse!

The St. Louis Downtown Airport, where I work, is a good stopping place for the Goodyear blimps when they are en route from one engagement to another. One time, the Houston-based Goodyear blimp *America* spent a few days at our airport for a promotion. Before the flight, its pilot offered two lucky people a couple of the blimp's extra seats. A coworker and I were lucky to be included, and during the flight, the pilot gave all of the passengers an opportunity to fly. As if Cupid had punctured my heart with his arrow, I was instantly and totally in love with this new facet of aviation. With the goal of applying for a job as a blimp pilot, I soon obtained my multi-engine rating. I continued to be enthralled by airships, such as blimps, and so with letters and phone calls, I stayed in touch with people I knew at Goodyear in Akron, Ohio.

Should I pursue a job as a blimp pilot, I wondered? Blimp pilots were on the road six months out of the year, and Goodyear didn't maintain a base near St. Louis. I would have less job security and no retirement plan. Still, I was attracted to the idea. While shopping one day, I saw a card with an embroidered message mounted on a bright red mat. It said, "All Things Are Sweetened by Risk." Yes, that was exactly true. I bought the card, put it in a red frame and made it my new motto.

Finally, I was offered an interview for a job opening at the Goodyear Airship Base in Pompano Beach, Florida. I interviewed in Akron, Ohio, where Goodyear's headquarters are located. As the day passed, it became apparent to me that an underlying sexist attitude prevailed in the company: Girls don't fly blimps! But I was still determined to pursue my dream, even if it meant having to cope with sexist attitudes.

I learned several weeks after the interview that I didn't get the job. The company suggested that I apply for a pilot position for a new aircraft that was currently under construction, saying that it was lighter and didn't require as much "strength" to fly.

When that door shut, I decided to become a flight instructor, and before I knew it, I had more students than I could handle. I worked seven days a week, along with my duties at the tower, and only had a day off when the weather was poor and no one could fly. This was my schedule for the next five years, and despite the hectic hours, I loved it.

On Memorial Day 1995, I woke up with a little numbness in my left knee. I thought I'd slept on it wrong and waited for it to go away. Not only did it continue to feel numb, but two days later my legs felt sensitive to the touch. So did my hair. I was feeling poorly, and by the end of the week, I was having difficulty going to the bathroom.

My doctor suggested that I had shingles; I felt deflated by his suggestion. My mom was still getting over a bout with shingles that had made her very uncomfortable for the past three months. I knew if I had shingles, I would be unable to work in the tower for the Oshkosh fly-in in August.

The annual Experimental Aircraft Association fly-in takes place in Oshkosh, Wisconsin, each summer. For one week at the end of July, this little airport in northern Wisconsin becomes busier than Chicago's O'Hare and hosts the widest variety of aircraft in the world. This is the aviation event all flying enthusiasts worldwide dream about, and most attend at least once. The best of the best, the cream of the crop, the pinnacle of controllers work in the tower during the event. I had applied to work in the tower every year during my thirteen years as an air traffic controller. Finally, in February 1995, I received the word: I was finally high enough on the seniority list and at last had been selected. During those four months, my flying buddies were getting used to my singsong "I'm going to Oshkosh! I'm going to Oshkosh!" They were jealous in a good-natured way, and I couldn't wait to go. Unfortunately, my first experience with multiple sclerosis would prevent my dream from coming true.

I met my doctor at the hospital after a few days of continuing bladder problems. He decided to admit me to the hospital to search for the problem. After eight days as an inpatient, the neurologist said he was pretty sure I had MS.

I went home to rethink how my days were going to play out. I had a hard time getting out of the workaday mind-set because work is what I do. The neurologist had told me that I could still live a full and productive life with MS. "Not as an air traffic controller and a flight instructor!" I countered. I had been wishing for a month off work with full pay and now my wish had come true. Unfortunately, I hadn't also wished for health and energy. Walking from the bathroom to the bedroom wore me out.

After six weeks, I was no longer off work at full pay. Having run out of sick leave and vacation time, I spent a few more weeks on leave without pay. Amazingly, what seemed to have such importance just a few months ago didn't matter much now in the grand scheme of things.

When I could barely walk in June, I refused to believe that I wouldn't be well enough to work in the tower at the Oshkosh fly-in at the end of July. Finally, I could deny it no more. I was forced to write a letter to my boss, relinquishing the prized temporary duty.

It wasn't much of a surprise when, shortly after, the Federal Aviation Administration sent me a certified letter telling me that I'd lost my medical certification, which meant that I could no longer work as a pilot or an air traffic controller.

I had been expecting this, but I wasn't prepared for the anger that followed. Aviation had been my life. I simply could not envision a future without it. So I came up with a plan: I was going to get my medical certification back.

I have always been the antithesis of what the world defines as a "normal girl." When I was younger, very few women were pilots or air traffic controllers, and teenagers seldom became pilots. This never deterred me from doing exactly what I wanted with my life. After I was diagnosed, my experiences in nonconformity would serve me well.

Being in an airplane is like being home to me. The sky is my address, the place where I feel most alive. When I'm flying, life's burdens are left behind. All of my negative feelings fall away. It's a palpable and tangible loosening of tension and pressure, and I become thoroughly focused on the task at hand. Which way is the wind blowing? I study the landscape beneath me: the red roof of a Pizza Hut, the long rows of crops planted in perfect lines. Each flight is unique, yet as comfortable and familiar as an old pair of sneakers. This is the feeling you get when you know where you belong.

Was the disease capable of rearranging my experience, my expertise? I didn't think so. What I know about flying is an inseparable part of me. When I sit, huddled in the second seat beside a student, I am focused on the airspeed, or the crosswind. Everything in the airplane is a fine balance of power settings, airplane angle, heading and course. There are moments when I become aware of my own knowledge and expertise about flying, and they leave me breathless. There is nothing I want more than to share what I do best with others.

By Labor Day, I was strong enough to return to work part-time, working on administrative duties for six hours a day. I had the full support of the union, which gave me several suggestions about how to get my medical certification back, and I also had a few ideas of my own. One day, my supervisor poked his head in the door of my small office and said, "The FAA picked the wrong woman to mess with!"

He was accurate. I hurdled every roadblock the FAA put in my way and awaited the next one with poise. When my manager expressed concern over whether I could work a full eight-hour day, I immediately requested my hours be changed from six to eight per day.

Still the FAA insisted I retire. The prospect of being broke with a 60 percent pay reduction did not appeal to me at all; I could hardly make ends meet on 100 percent pay. And I couldn't imagine the day when I'd land a plane for the last time, or give one last glance to the long runway from the tower.

The official retirement form arrived in the mail. On it were two boxes to be checked: I could check the "Okay, I'm outta here" box, or the "Hell no, I won't go" box. I marked the latter, automatically appealing the decision, and then prepared myself for battle.

I had my neurologist send a copy of my MRI scans to the FAA. I also sent a videotape of me at my dance class, to show my previous balance problems had improved.

Eventually, I was contacted by a doctor from the FAA who gave further suggestions; I made two more video-tapes in which I engaged in various physical and mental activities. I also sent more printed documentation. In the end, the FAA had three boxes of documentation to go through. I figured at some point, if nothing else, the FAA would say, "Just give her the darned medical back. We're sick of hearing from that Earhart woman!"

But the FAA countered by saying that the medication I was taking wasn't on the list of approved drugs. I knew there was no such list; when I pressed for a copy, the FAA simply restated the reasons for denying me my certification for reasons other than my medication.

Luckily, I had a pilot friend who also worked as an aviation medical examiner. Together we looked up the types of documentation required by the FAA to issue certifications to those with medical disorders; the FAA uses different tests and procedures depending on the medical condition. Because of the unpredictability of neurological disorders, each case was handled individually.

Ten months after I was diagnosed, I jumped the final hurdle and was reissued a medical certificate that would allow me to fly, work as a flight instructor and control air traffic. I even received a letter from the FAA's head flight surgeon commending me on the use of video in documenting my appeal. When some of the regular pilots, who knew me from my thirteen years in the tower, heard me on the radio again, I was universally congratulated and welcomed back. No one was as happy to be back as I was.

Over the past few years, I have been in contact with other pilots and air traffic controllers who have been diagnosed with MS. Sometimes the union refers a newly diagnosed controller to me, or someone will see my name listed in the membership directory of Women in Aviation International. I realize the importance of helping others, since I didn't have anyone before me setting a precedent. My struggle has helped the pilots and controllers with MS who have·followed behind me. They have forged their own trails, and in turn their efforts have helped me.

I hope someday to create a Web site providing

information and success stories specifically geared toward pilots and controllers with MS. Because our numbers are relatively few—the total number of pilots flying with neurological disorders is fewer than the number of pilots flying with pacemakers—a network of mutual support is needed all the more. In the meantime, I have become involved in Wheelchairs on Wings, a charitable organization that provides scholarships to disabled people to help them earn their pilot's licenses. The program took root in the United Kingdom, and we hope to expand it someday to the United States.

It has been five years since my diagnosis. I still have the job that I love, and I'm moving the metal with the best of them. I speak to aviation groups, hoping to encourage and inspire others with my story. I enjoy crossing paths with pilots; I am energized by their enthusiasm and the high regard in which they seem to hold me. I am also encouraging other women to take up flying, as a career or as a hobby.

The Aero Club has asked me to return more actively as an instructor, and although I'd like to, the window in which I can fly has narrowed somewhat because of the heat and humidity of St. Louis summers; heat and MS have never been friends. But during the winter months, you can find me on the runway, getting ready for flight. All thoughts of disease are left beneath me as we leave the ground; there is nothing in my life at that moment except for that flight, the inextricable roar of the engine, the feeling of freedom in the air. I think this is what is meant by living in the moment.

In each and every life, there are challenges. You can choose to let the challenges defeat you, or you can defeat the challenges. The question to ask yourself is "What do I choose? What do I want for myself?

Life is good, but I'd still like to fly a blimp.

DIANE EARHART *is an air traffic controller in the St. Louis, Missouri area, and a multi-engine-rated pilot and flight instructor. In January 1999, she was named the Aviation Safety Counselor of the Year for the St. Louis district. Earhart started a peer support group in her community for others living with MS, and devotes time to volunteering for the local National MS Society chapter. In 1999, she was selected by the National Multiple Sclerosis Society Gateway Area Chapter to receive the Individual Achievement of the Year award. She enjoys traveling both in the United States and abroad; most recently, she traveled to Britain to speak at a pilots' conference. She also participates in fund-raising for Wheelchairs on Wings, a charitable organization that provides scholarships to disabled people to obtain a pilot's license. She also enjoys dancing in an adult jazz and ballet class. Your e-mail messages are welcome at* Earhart500@aol.com, *and her speaking schedule is available at* www.aviationhumour.co.uk/diane.htm.

7

RECLAIMING OUR PAST

Eric Simons

Climbing is the cruelest sport, a beckoning siren, sweetly calling out the treacherous poetry of the hills and crags. "In the mountains, there you feel free," it intones, drawing us inexorably into the severe and unforgiving beauty of a vertical world devoid of the green and bustle of life: the wasteland.

I remember my first taste of this opiate more than three decades ago, sitting under an arching willow, reading a book my oldest brother had just checked out of the public library: *Rock Climbers in Action in Snowdonia*. The black-and-white photographs of tweed-clad climbers testing their mettle among the barren, rugged moors of Wales lured me in, firing my boyhood fantasies to brilliant incandescence. Simian proclivities awakened that day, and I was launched into a life on the rocks.

Climbing has taught me many lessons. It has taught me the joy and peace of simplicity and focus. It has taught me the wonder of detail and small pleasures. It has taught me to think big, but to step carefully. It has taught me to pierce the veil of fear, and to believe in the fact that I am a survivor. It has taught me that when push comes to shove, I am the only one responsible for myself. This lesson proved equally invaluable when I was diagnosed with MS.

> I REALIZED I WAS A WELL OF POTENTIAL AND THAT MS HAD SIMPLY ALTERED MY MIX, SHUTTING OFF SOME POTENTIALITIES, BUT OPENING UP A WHOLE RAFT OF OTHERS.

I have always questioned my toughness, but have found faith in my ability to sniff out and avoid serious danger, or to extricate myself when the danger is unavoidable. In many cases, my timidity has caused me to back off when others might have forged ahead, something I regret at times. Then again, I am still here and many of those hardier, or possibly foolhardy, climbers are not.

Being a fence-sitter, with the fire of my passions often quelled by social obligations and parental expectations, I have bounced between climbing epics and responsibility. After graduating from college in Connecticut, I hit upon the bright idea of using my climbing talents to become a tree surgeon, only to have that fire doused by my parents' disapproval and their insistence that I enter a more respectable profession. They felt the expense and prestige of my private university education, as well as my potential, deserved more than the image of a scruffy monkey man hacking away at tree limbs in doctors' and lawyers' backyards.

And so, after a year of aimless work at nuclear laboratories, punctuated by weekends on the rocks in New Paltz, New York, I settled on law school, an option I loathed, because so many pompous Type A people I knew were obsessively ensconced in law libraries throughout the Northeast, hiding key cases from their moot court opponents and developing pasty complexions. I had caved in to parental pressure reluctantly, but in so doing, I acquiesced to a value system I had partially internalized. Remarkably, like water seeking the easiest path to the sea, I was now coursing unconsciously toward fulfillment.

After a few months, the East Coast educational myopia, as well as my parents' desperate attempts to find me a "nice New York girl," gave way to my desire to migrate west into the heart of the mountains. I transferred to the

University of Denver College of Law to finish my legal education, though I really moved to climb.

Moving to Boulder, Colorado, felt like moving home. Living in New York had been frantic, with energy crackling from every storefront, the clotted traffic and the endless apartments stacked like a Gothic cordwood nightmare. While living in Manhattan, I sought solitude by venturing into Central Park during blizzards, reasoning that it was too cold even for the muggers. I would sit in the snow, swathed in all of my warmest down gear, savoring the quiet, the calm and the cool wet of the snowflakes on my eyelashes. The dark hulks of the buildings were only muted shadows beyond a wall of snow. In Boulder, there was more quiet and solitude at the end of my block than you could stuff into ten thousand Central Parks.

My wife claims we met in law school; I claim we met at a bar. Both true, but the fact is, our first words were exchanged at the RTD bus stop in front of Duffy's Bar in downtown Denver while waiting for the regional bus to whisk us back to Boulder after class on Tuesday and Thursday nights. Though I had never seen her before, she apparently had noticed my bushy hair, chin-strap beard and lightning-bolt earring flashing in the morning sun while riding the bus.

While my parents had been conspiring to find me that nice "New York girl," I had been dreaming of my "country girl," a natural beauty with minimal make-up, laser-sharp intelligence and small-town sensibilities: someone who would share my love of the outdoors and solitude, and especially, someone who would tolerate my fanaticism for climbing. Though Linnea was six years older than me, I realized I had found my country girl: a beautiful, blue-eyed Swede from Glenwood Springs, Colorado, with long blonde hair, liberal tendencies, her own little yellow clapboard house, a wonderful raspberry patch in the garden and a gentle black dog named Axel, who was spoiled rotten.

I was enchanted by this lady and asked if I could move in with her. Linnea—older, wiser and weary from relationships that hadn't worked out—laid the gauntlet at my feet. She approved of the cohabitation on one condition: that we would get married. I had not planned on matrimonial ties until much later in life, and certainly not after only three weeks of courtship, but I doubted that I would ever find someone else like her. I agreed to her ultimatum, flowing into the arms of the woman who would be my one love and my life companion.

After the wedding, we spent our honeymoon backpacking in the Sierras, hiking along the fog-bound beaches and tidal pools at Point Reyes and climbing in Yosemite. Graduation came and went and we entered our respective careers: Linnea went to a large Denver law firm, and I to my philosophical antithesis, the oil industry. Being six years older, Linnea's biological clock chimed steadily, demanding that something be done, and I found myself a father at the age of twenty-seven, wondering how to juggle climbing and diapers.

Our little family was launched, followed in 1985 by the adoption of Marc, a beautiful boy of mixed race from the city of Fortaleza on the northern coast of Brazil. Noah, our surprise third son, was born in 1988 and, as we had reached our goal of two children born to us and one adopted, I went under the knife, snipped to sterility in a short and sore twenty minutes. Climbing remained a constant, though Linnea was never happy when I plunked the kid down in the portable playpen at the base of a climb, asking the occasional passerby to check on him while I climbed, ready to rappel down if a bottle or diaper change were needed.

Jobs came and went, the boys grew—and grew louder— as we dubbed ourselves the Loud Family, and I found myself, in 1993, doing laundry, volunteering in the schools, cleaning toilets and cooking dinner, as Linnea churned away in the legal department of US West. The domestic life took a little getting used to—even for a liberated American male such as myself. My latest oil venture had soured: After eighteen months as the entrepreneurial president of my own little oil and real estate development company in Russia and Kazakhstan, I came home, having drained far too much of our savings, tail between my legs, chastened by my unsuccessful attempt to become a multimillionaire.

Though my culinary ineptitude was turning into culinary aptitude, domesticity gave way to career. I decided to acquire another graduate degree, and entered the University of Denver Environmental Policy and Management Master's Program, hoping to hire myself out to the extractive industries as an environmental compliance consultant. For the first time in my long school career, I actually learned how to study and apply myself, making the sacrifices I had been unwilling to make before in pursuit of education and grades. This time I was successful and graduated in the summer of 1995 at the top of my class, but I found that the market had turned and work was scarce.

Rock 'n' roll lyrics can provide a poetic crystallizing of life's flow into easily digestible platitudes. The Grateful Dead wrote, "When life looks like easy street, there is danger at your door," while Joni Mitchell sang, "Just when you think you've finally got it made, bad news comes knocking at your garden gate." Though not nabobs of negativity, the Dead and Joni recognized the inherent uncertainty in life, and the need to acknowledge the possibility of tragedy in the midst of plenty. Cotton Mather, as he sermonized to his parishioners in early New England, roared incessantly about how, without a moment's notice, the earth could open up and swallow you, carrying you away into the darkness for eternity.

In November 1995, I went climbing in Eldorado Canyon, seven miles south of my home. "Eldo" is one of the premier climbing lodestones in the United States, a narrow creek-carved canyon hemmed in by 600-foot red sandstone cliffs rising vertically from the boulder fields, streaked with yellow and green lichen, and swathed in hordes of acrobatic swallows.

My climbing buddy, Larry, and I decided on a Sunday climb of Long John Wall on a cliff named the West Ridge. Long John was a beautiful and easy climb, but steep, forcing us to crane our necks, as we watched each other lead our respective portions of the route. It was a perfect late fall day, full of quiet expectation and a sense of being poised on the cusp, balanced between the lazy warmth of the Indian summer and the heartless winds of winter.

I drove home sated, but as with some pleasant climbs, there was a dark lining to this silver cloud. I had developed a stiff neck on Long John and spent the evening rubbing the knotted muscles in my neck and upper back while ingesting vitamin "I," known to the general nonathletic public as ibuprofen.

Sleep has been called the "little death," a time of vulnerability when we dissolve, the floodgates of the unconscious thrown open and the demons hovering, waiting to pierce any chink in the armor. Though sleep is also a time of renewal, it is no wonder we pull the covers up, wear our lucky pajamas and wait anxiously for the bright dawn. That night, while asleep after climbing Long John Wall, something happened to me—something completely unexpected and unwelcome that would change my life forever.

I woke to find that I had no feeling on the right side of

my body from my neck to my toes. Incredulous, I stomped my right foot on the bathroom floor, pinched my right arm, ran my nails along the flesh of my belly, and stared at my image in the spotted mirror, trying to see if there was any visible sign of malady. As the panic gathered in my belly, I felt as if I'd woken to a dream within a dream, woken to find myself dangling from the end of a rope, with no idea how I'd gotten there and no idea how to extricate myself.

Ever the optimist, unwilling to acknowledge the potential seriousness of this new lack of sensation, I convinced myself that the numbness was probably the result of a pinched nerve, acquired while contorting my body on the climb. As I ate my breakfast, I told my wife that if the numbness didn't improve within two days, I'd go see the doctor. As my wife scurried to work and the kids scurried to school, I sat, trying to rationalize this sudden turn of events. I stared at my right hand, clutching the handle of my "I'm out of the loop and that's the way I like it!" mug, sensation dulled, as if I were wearing gloves. The world, roiling with life, blithely rolled on, oblivious to this tectonic shift in my kingdom. Numb, I continued with my daily rituals, brushing my teeth, folding laundry, making phone calls and tapping away at the keyboard as my tactile world receded. I had no alternative; I helplessly watched my body betray me.

By the following morning, the fantasy of improvement had dissipated with the prior night's dreams. Despite wishful thinking, the numbness had not retreated, but had staged another assault, and I no longer had any feeling in my body from the neck down. The acid of panic churned in my stomach as I stood in front of the mirror, pinching and poking both sides of my body and stomping both feet on the cool floor tiles. Nothing. No sensation at all, though my neck and head seemed to be unaffected. My wife's occasional comment about my being numb from the neck up careened through my brain, as I realized I'd fooled her this time and had gone the other way. I was beginning to feel as if I were climbing far from the safety of protection, while my handholds crumbled beneath my fingers and my partner watched helplessly in the distance. I had such a long, long way to fall.

After everyone had left, I decided to call the doctor and arranged to see him the next day. I then walked a block and a half to Foothill Elementary School, still mobile, but unable to feel my clothing or the coolness of the November air. I was becoming disembodied, a consciousness only remotely connected to the physical form that had housed it for forty years. I had turned robotic, a puppet master directing my body's stiff movements from a distance. My volunteer duties in Marc's fourth-grade classroom were carried out carefully, as I struggled to maintain a facade of normalcy.

"Well, these symptoms are troubling, Eric, but I really think you should go home and rest for awhile. If they don't go away, call me. Often, these sorts of things can be caused by emotions."

I sat on the examination table in my doctor's office, the sterile paper crinkling beneath me, as I shifted awkwardly, not certain whether I had heard him correctly. My doctor leaned against the counter in the examination room at the Boulder Medical Center, his narrow pinched face radiating concern beneath wisps of sparse gray hair and a forehead mottled by brown age spots. I had just been told that my symptoms were psychosomatic, dismissed as a self-inflicted problem caused by hypochondriacally induced hysteria. An image of the fainting ladies of the late nineteenth century, overly tight corsets squeezing the consciousness from their bodies, flitted through my mind. That image would stay with me, as two years later, I would meet a woman in a wheelchair who had been told by her doctor when her MS symptoms first appeared that her real problem was that her jeans were too tight.

"I can't believe these symptoms are psychosomatic," I said. "I don't manifest my emotional problems physically. This isn't just a minor complaint. I can't feel a thing."

"Still, I think you should rest and see how this progresses."

Medical stonewalling won the day and I left, driving the six blocks to my home slowly, deflated and frustrated. Maybe I could have been a more aggressive advocate of my cause. Maybe I could have insisted that my doctor conduct a more thorough examination, or refer me to another physician who would actually listen to my tale of woe. As with millions of other patients, I didn't, because I had been indoctrinated to defer to the medical profession in matters of health care. I didn't, because I was so emotionally drained by my numbness that I couldn't muster the energy to fight the professional intransigence.

That afternoon, true to my nature, I wallowed in self-pity, frustration and confusion. The wallowing gave way to resolve, and just before dinner, I called my brother Steven, a doctor in Brooklyn, to ask for his advice. Predictably, but gratifyingly, he agreed that my symptoms deserved closer attention and encouraged me to contact my doctor again. The next day, my doctor, faced with my annoying insistence, acquiesced and agreed to make an appointment for me with a neurologist. Our behemoth managed-care system, however, raised its numerous defenses and blocked immediate treatment. I left the Boulder Medical Center later, card in hand, reminding me of my appointment in two weeks with the only local neurologist who was "on network."

As the weekend approached my numbness deepened, my right arm became paralyzed, and I became exasperated by the lack of immediate medical care for my worsening condition. The fingers of my right hand curved in, clawlike, and I began stashing my right hand in my jeans pocket in order to control this limb that no longer responded to my commands. I found all attempts to use my hand were fruitless, as it had turned into an insensate block of wood. I was forced to begin the slow and difficult process of learning to use my left hand instead. I was reluctantly learning that necessity is, indeed, the mother of invention.

Saturday afternoon before Thanksgiving, I lay in bed, exhausted from the physical and emotional drain of my undiagnosed illness, looking out the bay window toward the mountains two blocks from my house, now turned brown beneath the weak blue of the November sky. I gazed longingly at the hills, wondering whether I would ever be able to immerse myself in them again, smelling the mustiness of the rain-soaked dust, or feeling the creak of my knees as I pounded up the rocky trails.

Everyone with a neurological disease should have a neurologist for a neighbor. As I looked out toward the hills, I saw my wife talking with our neighbor Dr. Bob, the neurologist. She stood beneath the blue spruce, arms crossed over her pile jacket, protection against the chill of the afternoon. I closed my eyes and woke several minutes later to find Dr. Bob and my wife standing next to the bed. The ensuing brief examination, the gentle pokes and prods and testing of my reflexes, evoked a greater and more rapid response from Bob than a month of such evaluations would have from my own physician.

Alarmed by my sorry condition, Bob returned to his house and, in stark contrast to the misguided recalcitrance of my own physician, arranged for me to have an

MRI of my neck that evening. Although I would have preferred going out to dinner and a movie with my wife, while tightly wrapped in the cool embrace of modern medical technology, I welcomed the MRI's symphonic cacophony of staccato clicks and wrenching groans.

Sunday morning after the MRI, another neurologist called to inform me that the MRI had detected a large lesion on my spinal cord in my neck in the area of the C3 vertebra. I was advised to check into the hospital that morning for a three-day visit. With a small bag containing a change of clothes and some toiletries, I checked in, feeling like a child who senses that danger is imminent but, due to inexperience, is confused and wholly reliant upon the adults in his life to make the decisions and to usher him down the path to safety.

My three days in the hospital during Thanksgiving week are now a blur, but resulted in a diagnosis of MS, a disease that was a mystery to me at the time. In my confusion, I imagined joining Jerry Lewis on his telethons, until one of the nurses gently told me that Jerry's kids had muscular dystrophy, a completely different Gordian knot.

MS, MD, whatever. They both sucked. With my paradigm irrevocably shifted, I stumbled home from the hospital to the protective herd of family, was ushered to my bedroom, given my wife's side of the bed (talk about paradigm shifts) and hooked up to the home-health-care-intravenous-setup that would be my constant companion for the next three days. Shades drawn, door mostly closed, light softening the space, the room became the archetypal haven for the sick, as my family periodically tromped upstairs to sit with me, check my tubes and make quiet small talk.

Thanksgiving was difficult, as I sat at the table next to my wife, unsteady in my chair and unable to cut my food because my right arm had descended into paralysis. Sitting around the cornucopia during our favorite holiday, my family, including my parents and my brother and his family, were subdued in awkward silence, as they struggled to fashion an acceptably normal conversation in the presence of someone so obviously a mess.

"Sure, everything's fine," I wanted to say, "though it's going to be damn hard traveling in India when I'm going to have to wipe *and* eat with the left hand!" Instead, I just stared at the turkey on the platter feeling real brotherhood with a piece of poultry, as I thought about how we both had just gotten the raw end of the deal.

By this point, I had a veritable laundry list of MS symptoms, including total lack of sensation from my neck down, paralysis of my right arm, vertigo, banded abdominal pain, severe headaches and very odd pressure sensations in my head, making me feel like the protagonist in the movie *American Werewolf in London* as his face erupted forward to form a snarling hairy snout. MS may be the ultimate existential neurological disease; it disrupts our sense of complacency and self with a plethora of capriciously shifting symptoms, predictably unpredictable. It is an intensely emotional disease, not just because the ravaged sections of our central nervous systems may actually produce chemically induced depression, but because it rips away our emotional foundations, relentlessly assaulting us with our fragile nature and forcing us to take a good hard look at who we are.

I was devastated by the diagnosis. In one fell swoop, I had been metamorphosed from the hale and hardy mountaineer, the provider, the "rock" of the family, into an invalid requiring assistance with almost everything. As a man with a strong independent streak, this was difficult because asking for help, let alone really needing it, was an anathema. I was the one who always helped everyone else. Still, I accepted the help because I really had no choice. MS had made it very difficult for me to accomplish many basic daily functions. Contributing to my begrudging acceptance of the new paradigm was a childhood, tinged by uncertainty and pregnant with change, that had made me resilient and flexible enough to roll with the blows. In addition, my periodic forays into domesticity while between jobs had opened my eyes to realities other than being a 17th Street "suit." While I wanted to be the strong oak, it was the spirit of the grass that allowed me to weather the intense storm that was blowing through me.

The day after finishing the oral prednisone taper down, I began to run a fever, which was then diagnosed at the local medical center as the flu. After all, it was flu season and I did have a fever. Five days of lying in bed with a high fever, popping Tylenol, brought me to the point where I could barely raise myself off the pillow. Sensing that something was really wrong and that this was unlike any bout with the flu I had ever had, I asked Linnea to take me to see my doctor. He examined me briefly, and informed us that I needed to check into the hospital immediately. We drove the half block across Broadway, and I was loaded into a wheelchair to be taken to my room in the cancer ward at the hospital.

Though I generally don't cleave to this idea, sometimes ignorance really is bliss. Though I can't say that I was blissed out that December 6 in 1995, I was lucky not to have been privy to a brief conversation my doctor had with Linnea in a small patient counseling room across the hall from my room. While acknowledging inadequate information, my doctor solemnly told Linnea that my condition appeared to be the result of extremely advanced pancreatic cancer, that I probably would not make it through the night and that she should start making "preparations" for my death.

The next morning, fortunately, I was still alive. In their attempt to identify the cause of my illness, the doctors began a battery of tests. By early afternoon, the CAT scan had been completed and reviewed by a bevy of doctors, who then appeared at my door to give me the good news.

"The good news, Eric, is that we can't find any cancer. The bad news, however, is that you're dying and we haven't a clue as to why."

Unfortunately, this second illness, which was unrelated to MS, was never conclusively diagnosed, much to my dismay, as well as that of the attending physicians. Apparently, several of my systems were shutting down, subjecting me to grave risk.

I was in the hospital for nine days, six of those semi comatose, lying in my small room, occasionally waking to see one or another of my family sitting quietly at the foot of my bed, glumly watching me and waiting for some improvement. I am thankful for the support of my family during this time, because I was unable to advocate for myself. In particular, my wife and my mother, who is a physician, rode herd on the medical staff to make sure that everything that could be done was done. I am also thankful for the wonderfully compassionate, gentle and attentive care given by the nurses, whose daily ministrations softened the frightening reality of what was happening to me.

While conscious, dreadfully aware that something was draining the life from my body, and knowing that death was only a click away, I struggled to come to grips with the concept of dying at the ripe young age of forty. I felt conflicted: on the one hand wanting to rage against the dying of the light, and on the other, wishing for peace and the willingness to accept the inevitability of my death. Desperately rationalizing the quality of my forty years, my wife and my children, my climbs, my education and professional accomplishments, my legacy gave way to the tidal force of biology as the miracle of the double helix screamed from every cell.

We all search for the strength to sustain us in times of need and I searched, during my lucid moments, for that source of inspiration that would infuse me with the energy to survive. When the going gets tough, the tough go shopping, and I was shopping for something to anchor me. It is at these times that all the superfluous junk, the socially manufactured baggage, the personal idiosyncrasies get stripped away, and we are left with the essence of who we are. Kowtowing to the biological imperative, I found my essence, my purpose, my strength very clearly and very undeniably in one place: my children. I had to pull through, not so much for myself or my marriage, but for my three boys. As with all of our less aware, but equally instinctive friends in the animal world, I had to be there to provide for, to protect and to teach my children until they were able to fend for themselves. Grasping at my love for them and theirs for me, I fought, feeling like a sailor clinging to a life raft named Evan, Marc and Noah, as I was buffeted by the storm that wracked my body.

After nine days, the storm calmed and I returned home to my shaded bedroom—this time to my side of the bed—barely able to sit up for more than a minute at a time. I was stunned, in shock, feeling like a wildebeest standing helplessly in a *National Geographic* photo— eyes wide and empty, guts and life force pouring through

a rent in its belly as lions tear relentlessly at its vulnerability. Melodrama had become my reality. I think of this
period in my life as "The Hunkering Down," a time
when, with no real alternative, I focused on conserving
my resources. Much like huddling inside my sleeping
bag during the winter, preserving my spark of life against
the cold world, I concentrated on preserving my spark of
life against the illnesses that had devastated me.

My life consisted of lying in bed staring out the window,
watching dismal daytime television and waiting for the
onset of my daily seizures. As my family ministered to my
needs, an astounding number of friends, neighbors and
acquaintances stopped by to offer help, bring a home-
cooked meal, or assist with shuttling my two younger boys
to their various lessons and appointments. I learned that
we are bigger than ourselves, we are each part of a community, and the more we do for others, the more connected
and greater our lives will be. My years of community service and attentiveness to all the people in my life paid back
in spades, and I was buoyed upward on an ocean of love.

As I lay staring out my window, past my yard and
gazebo to the mountains, I began to actively explore the
reality of my new life and the consequences of my illness,
rather than just reacting to the latest crisis. At this time my
symptoms had stabilized, becoming more predictable and
allowing me to reflect on my situation—a luxury I had
not had while living the panicked life, wondering what
new terror would visit me like a wraith out of the dark.

My thoughts wandered to all of the downtrodden and afflicted, seeking solace and instruction in the fact that countless others had endured equal or worse and that they had survived and sometimes thrived. I was doing my best to personify the platitude "Misery loves company," knowing that I would always be topped in the one-upmanship of the miserable, but knowing also that I could now consider myself a solid member of the chorus. I thought about people enduring the horror of the "killing fields" of Cambodia, the dingy gray death trap of Bosnia, the starvation of AIDS-wracked Africa. Then I turned to individuals like Stephen Hawking—ALS having left his body barely functional while his mind is so vibrant and brilliant that he is counted among the giants of modern physics. I knew I would never achieve what Stephen Hawking has, but I hoped to contribute in some way.

During "The Hunkering Down," I also reconnected with climbing. Though I couldn't traipse through the hills, I remembered the lessons I had learned from years stuck to vertical rock faces. Though climbers are some-times seen as odd troglodytes who climb rocks, sleep under rocks and whose heads are full of rocks, we are, by nature, philosophical. In my rambling, I came to see that climbing requires certain attributes that are uniquely applicable to overcoming obstacles of all kinds. To climb and survive you must realistically assess your strengths and weaknesses. To climb, you must set lofty goals but be able to break those dreams down into smaller achievable segments. To climb, you must exhibit persistence and perseverance in the face of difficult conditions. To climb, you must become accepting of and adept at the use of tools. To climb, you must recognize that fear is always present, but that you can negotiate with it, manage it so that it doesn't prevent you from achieving your goals, and even use it, like the canary in the coal mine, as a litmus test of rising panic whispering emphatically to you that this time, it really is okay to retreat.

Though I could barely climb out of bed in January 1996, let alone climb mountains, I began to set goals, because I felt that without them, I would stagnate, eventually embarking on an irreversible downward spiral. While looking out to the gazebo in the yard, I decided that I would do everything in my power—of which there was very little at that point—to achieve a full recovery from my exacerbation. The first step toward achieving that goal would be to walk out to the gazebo and watch my sons play. Because of MS and the second illness, my world had narrowed dramatically. I genuinely believed that if I could just toddle around the yard watching the kids, I could be happy for the rest of my life. I have a talent for underestimating.

Several days later, on a warm January day, I walked to the gazebo, watched the kids play and then staggered back to the house, exhausted, but elated. As I lay in my bed, again looking out the window, recovering from the foray to the gazebo, I felt my contentment erode as the old climbing genes began to reassert themselves. If I could walk to the gazebo, I wondered, maybe I could make it to the end of the block and back.

One small step led to another, and another.

As I sat resting in the snow in February 1999 at 22,550 feet above sea level, my oxygen-starved brain was caught in a feedback loop of lyrics from the Rolling Stones: "You can't always get what you want, but if you try sometimes you just might find you get what you need." I looked out over the panorama spread before me and thought about the panorama of my life with MS.

I had failed in my bid for the summit of the Argentinean mountain Aconcagua, fewer than 300 vertical feet above me, not because of my own physical frailty, but because of my partner's. In the six days since we had left basic camp, ferrying loads and moving our camps up the mountain, Jim had been very slow. I didn't complain because the slower the ascent, the less likely you are to develop altitude sickness. His pace also felt comfortable and quite leisurely to me. *One step, five breaths, one step, five breaths.* We had already seen some deaths on the mountain during our climb, and I had no interest in becoming another statistic.

While it is important to conserve energy at high altitude, pace matters. The slower your progress, the more likely you will be caught by external dangers such as storms. Speed must be balanced against the need to acclimatize properly. On our summit day, Jim was moving slowly, as usual. His dry, high-altitude cough, more like a bark, periodically punctuated the quiet as we followed a line of red spots in the snow, markers left previously by a climber whose every breath brought up blood-stained sputum. By 21,500 feet, Jim's coughs were bringing up blood and we stopped to rest and talk about his condition. There was no question about what Jim needed to do: He had to descend. The only question was whether I would descend with him, a course of action that I insisted upon. Jim, however, convinced me that he would be fine.

While I appreciated Jim's desire for me to summit, I was skeptical about the possibility of success, since it was quite late in the afternoon and the next 1,300 vertical feet would be quite taxing. I was already almost four hours behind my normal pace and would have to make up time if I was to stand at the top of South America. Nevertheless, the lure of the summit was strong and I set off at an accelerated pace, passing a delirious Polish woman and two other people whose brains were addled by the altitude. Surprisingly, for someone with MS, I felt fine—though tired—and was comforted by the fact that these other climbers, disabled by the scarcity of oxygen, were being attended to by their partners.

Climbing at this altitude was agonizing. Every two or three steps required several minutes of recovery. My strength was being siphoned off, one step at a time. By 5:00 P.M., I had reached my high point, just below the summit in a large rock- and snow-filled gully named the Canaleta. I shoved my ice axe in the snow and sat on my pack, having ascended 5,000 vertical feet in ten hours, realizing that I had run out of gas and worrying that if I pushed farther, I might run the risk of bringing on an MS exacerbation due to hyperexhaustion.

I had stumbled many times on the trail from my MS diagnosis to climbing Aconcagua, but had avoided out-right face plants by carefully selecting my projects and gently pushing the envelope, rather than taking the full-bore, damn-the-torpedoes approach. On the way, I learned to listen to my body and mind, stressing them to the point of growth and validation, but not overstressing to the point of collapse. Even so, I made mistakes, like the wonderful day ice climbing in late 1996, which, while fun and satisfying, resulted in two weeks of regres-sion. One step up and two steps back. Still, if we don't take risks and we don't push, we never learn our limits, a message I now spread as I criss cross the United States while giving motivational talks to MS sufferers.

A chronic illness can be a rude shock when first diag-nosed. Though unwelcome, it can, however, be a pivotal event affording growth, where comfort and complacency and myopia once ruled. Several months after my diagno-sis, I was having a haircut when my barber, a slightly effeminate, tattooed ex-sailor, biker, and father of two, said, with regard to my MS, "One door may close, but another will open."

At another time, I may have passed this off as cliché and responded with an off-color joke, but the statement struck me, engendering an incongruous epiphany in the barber's chair. It reminded me that, as chairman of a charitable foundation providing grants to people with MS, I am constantly delighted to find people with spunk and grit, drawing upon their hidden strengths to live fulfilling lives despite their disabilities. As Terry combed and snipped, I realized that I was a well of potential and that MS had simply altered my mix, shutting off some potentialities, but opening up a whole raft of others. I had to take personal responsibility and dip deep into that well—drawing upon old strengths while finding new ones.

To a large extent, we are governed by the pleasure principle in its myriad manifestations. While rock climbing may seem distinctly unpleasant to many, it was one of my joys. Now that the door to this obsession was no longer wide open, I searched for another path to the pleasure and freedom of the hills; I found it in less technical, but equally magnificent mountains. Looking forward, I think that if I am no longer able to be a happy hiker above the mountain stream, I will be a wheeled warrior on the accessible trails, finding my joy wherever I can, and trying my best not to run anyone over.

Sated by a small snack of nuts and raisins, I gazed out from the Canaleta at the Andes and felt tears well up, as the music running through my brain switched tracks from the Stones to the Allman Brothers. The raw dark intensity of the song *Whippin' Post* and the refrain "Sometimes I feel . . . like I've been tied to the whippin' post" personified the worst of my times with MS, dredging up memories of despair and physical ruin. I often used *Whippin' Post* as a key to unlock the emotional tidal wave associated with that period, because the depth of the emotion was something I craved. It gave me the opportunity to give thanks for what I had been able to accomplish.

I remembered calling the National MS Society in January 1996 to ask what I could do to fight this disease. I was forced to listen to a cheery voice on the other end of the line telling me, "It's truly a wonderful time to be diagnosed with MS!" If I had a cast-iron skillet, I would have beaned her.

In the ensuing years, I came to realize that what she had said was true, and that one of the cornerstones of my recovery—one of the foundations for my climb of Aconcagua—was interferon therapy, which had become commercially available in the last few years. Such drugs, along with the enormous quantity of current research, give all of us with MS hope and a tool to combat the disease. It is incumbent upon all of us with MS to use every tool at our disposal, to make our lives more fulfilling for ourselves and for our friends and family.

So I grabbed one of my tools, my ice axe, and, bracing myself, stood up, weary from the ascent and not looking forward to the long descent. With my eye's finger, I traced the numerous aesthetic routes on the adjoining peaks, beckoning me like a bevy of salacious sirens. In that exposed realm of rock and snow, I realized that it was best not to hide from the disease, but to accept it, embrace it, learn from it and move on. I pulled the ice axe out of the snow and started to plunge—stepping down: back to Jim, back to my tent at Nido de Condores, back to my family, back to my advocacy work in the MS community and back to the start of yet another climb.

ERIC SIMONS lives in Boulder, Colorado, with his wife, Linnea, sons Marc and Noah, and his dog Sabakah. His oldest son, Evan, attends the University of Colorado at Boulder. Eric has been an avid rock climber and mountaineer since the early 1970s, a passion that prompted his move from the Northeast to Colorado in 1979. Trained as a lawyer, this former oil-industry executive now dedicates much of his time to helping others with MS. Eric travels extensively around the United States giving motivational talks. He is also chairman of an MS-related charitable foundation, and he works closely with other MS-related nonprofit organizations. Eric continues to find joy climbing mountains in Colorado and around the world.

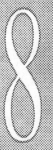

LIVING ONE DAY AT A TIME

Dean Kramer

MY FRIENDS, THE ASSISTIVE DEVICES

Over the past year, as my MS has moved deeper into secondary-progressive territory, several assistive devices have come into my life. It would sound more proactive to say "I chose several assistive devices." Technically, I did *choose* them, but I didn't want to have to choose them. I didn't want them at all. Even when I agreed I ought to have one of them, I felt ashamed of them. They made me visible as a disabled person, someone

I did not want to be—a "me" I could not imagine loving. They are, in order of their appearance in my life, a pair of trekking poles; a shower bench; an electric scooter; a lightweight, folding, manual wheelchair; a stairlift; and a wheelchair-accessible van equipped with hand controls.

What a process it has been getting to know and love them. In each case, I have, at first, had to leave them sitting unused awhile, letting myself get used to the idea of their presence in my life, my physical space, my consciousness. And then I'd use one of them—tentatively. I'd wonder, "Do I really *need* this?" Sometimes I'd say, "I don't really need one of these." But, inside, I knew I did.

> IF YOU WANT TO LEARN, AS MANY SPIRITUAL TEACHERS SUGGEST, THAT NOTHING IS TOTALLY YOURS TO CONTROL, [MS] IS A SUBJECT TO PRACTICE.

Over the weeks of continued residence in my home, each object, in turn, would get more and more use. It's second nature now to use the ones I've lived with longest, and the others are gradually making their way toward becoming a part of me, replacements for parts of me I can no longer rely upon.

I've always had a tendency toward anthropomorphism

regarding inanimate objects. Perhaps it was a premonition of becoming something of an inanimate object myself one day. Also, I have a mother who believed that furniture had opinions; that some sofas, for example, hated to be sat upon by certain objectionable people. Since the furnishings had no voices of their own, it was up to mother to interpret and speak for them. Leaving aside the question of the appropriateness of her remarks, I came into adulthood with the *feeling* that objects had feelings, that through use and over time one developed a relationship with the things in one's life. As my MS has worsened, I have become more and more dependent on objects. I depend on them to do what they were designed to do. I am more likely to be left helpless if they don't do what they were designed to do, since my body offers less and less latitude.

I find myself becoming friends with each of my assistive devices. I am learning their ways: the little squeak the trekking poles make, a quiet hum from the stairlift, which object likes to be greased (the stairlift) versus which ones like to be swept free of crumbs or polished. Knowing how these devices work, using and caring for them, are ways of putting out "good energy," certainly for their benefit and, as a result, on my own behalf as well. My caring attentions are repaid by their functioning smoothly (or by my noticing when they may not). And if *they* function smoothly, *I* function more smoothly than I otherwise could.

We live in a society, and at a time, when much attention is paid to the body. We are expected to care for and decorate our bodies. We are judged on the basis of how we appear measured against a standard of strength and beauty that I, at least, could not have matched even before MS, and certainly not since. These assistive devices of mine substitute on all sorts of levels for my own body's failing nervous system. They make a big difference as to how I look, what I can do and how I perceive myself.

These devices extend my boundaries inside and out. Tending them is tending me. Learning their workings teaches me about myself and stretches my mind. In accepting them, I am more able to accept myself. Coming to love them, I am really, finally, coming to love myself.

Together, these friends and I bring to mind the paradigm of person and tool: the cowboy and his trusty steed, the blind woman and her sensitive and intuitive guide dog, me and my van the "Moon Camel."

Yes, I think so.

BECAUSE IT'S THERE

I guess it's human nature for people to project their conflicts about being disabled onto physical obstacles, and then to focus on getting past them (or to retreat into depression because of them). So many of us write of "saving the farm," "climbing the mountain," "doing what it takes to get the job done."

What interests me is not whether one finally "wins," but how one *thinks* about the situation, how one decides who to *be*. When the ship is sinking, how do people decide what to keep, what to discard? Who confirms that our choices for survival are "right"?

The choice is often stated like this: "Do I sit around feeling sorry for myself, or go climb Mount Everest?"— a very either-or way of looking at things. Nevertheless...

I went to a party last night, held on the grounds of an "intentional community." You couldn't have designed a less accessible place for a physically disabled person if you'd set out to do so purposely. The party was held in a huge old mill that loomed at the end of a quarter-mile-long private drive. Many of the party-goers had parked on the verges of that drive and could be seen hiking with dogged cheer toward the mill. Though it was dusk and I couldn't be certain, I imagined the guests bearing their potluck offerings.

The party is a monthly event that rotates from location to location, depending on who has offered to host it. This was the first time it had been held in this location. The party is known for its wonderful variety of mainly vegetarian foods. And I, who had not eaten since breakfast, was looking forward to dinner.

I also knew that the community holding the party on this night tended toward very bland, vegan cooking (baked turnips with tempeh crumbles comes, unfortunately, to mind). But hungry as I was, I observed the arriving guests with anticipation of tastier fare.

My companion and I drove right up to the building, and backed into a parking space not far from the door. One of the owners appeared immediately and, as she began to remonstrate with us for taking a resident's parking space, I called out gaily, "But . . . I thought this was handicapped parking!" She swallowed her ire and said with instant political correctness, "Oh, right! Yes, that's right! Fine!" So I walked slowly with my stick over the rough and buckled driveway paving, clambered over a millstone set as a step and walked up three more slippery wooden steps to the door.

To my dismay, I found that the party was confined to the second floor, up a steep, narrow and uneven staircase with a rickety handrail. "Oh, dear," I said, not at all sure I could climb the stairs. The woman who'd just had her consciousness raised about handicapped parking told me that if I could not climb the stairs I might walk back down the driveway an eighth of a mile or so, and then up a shrub-covered, gradually rising hill (another eighth of a mile or so, and in darkness) to an entrance directly onto the second floor of the mill. When she saw my incredulous expression, she suggested that perhaps I could be driven back to the point where I'd need to begin climbing the dark and stairless hill. She presented these as serious alternatives. I did not burst out laughing in her face. After many years in psychotherapy, I am no longer given to such socially inappropriate behavior.

There I was, confronted by an external obstacle (the stairs, not the woman). And I had to make a choice. I could go back home and sit around feeling sorry for myself, or I could climb my own private Mount Everest. A fierce determination arose within me, a voice that said, "You go, girl, you came here to party!" So I climbed. I climbed, imagining the satisfying meal to be had once I reached the top. I climbed, carefully placing my feet and keeping a death grip on the trembling handrail as it threatened to pull out of the wall, and thinking of the delicious hot dishes awaiting me. And, through my own effort, undaunted, I reached the second floor of the old mill.

And here is what I found: On the floor of the dimly lit room, by a table laden with eating utensils, was a white plastic bucket of the sort used for house painting. Now, mind you, I was not wearing my reading glasses; and in the low light, with MS-related visual problems, things were a bit of a blur at that distance. But I swear it was filled with salad. Salad, in a bucket, on the floor. I asked a woman of my acquaintance if this was, in fact, a bucket of salad on the floor and, if so, were we meant to eat it? She hushed me and looked around warily—embarrassed, I suppose, that someone might have heard my query. Speaking in a very quiet voice, she opined that she wasn't at all sure exactly what it was and felt perhaps we'd best ignore it. That was not a problem.

What was a problem was the floor itself. It was very uneven: The old floorboards had warped and bowed, and small scatter rugs bunched menacingly underfoot, increasing my chances of falling. Additionally, since people often "don't see" the disabled, I had to steer clumsily around more swiftly and heedlessly mobile guests, muttering "Excuse me" and "So sorry" as I lurched and bumped. But driven by intrepid stubbornness and an empty stomach, I made my way to the food table.

I was carrying one of the many old china dishes that had been put out for guests to use. I had tried to choose a particularly ugly pattern from the variety of choices so that when (inevitably) at some point during the festivities I stumbled and it slipped from my MS-y hands and smashed to pieces, nobody would miss the plate too much.

You will think I am making this next part up, or heavily editing the truth, but that isn't the case. When I finally reached the food table, metaphoric summit of all my efforts, I found the following: a plate of blackberries, a plate containing overly toasted and dried-out triangles of pita bread near the crusted remains of what had been a bowl of hummus, and a plate containing raw (I mean cold and totally uncooked) tempeh. Nowhere in evidence were the wonderful covered-dish entrées my imagination had fed upon as I hauled my resisting body up the stairs, the creations I'd dreamed my way toward, the recipes that had inspired me to spit in the eye of misfortune and had kept me climbing, despite danger and disability, to the second floor of the old mill. There were only these few things.

I am more aware now—more than ever before—that our delusions are sometimes all we have to keep us going. One projects conflict about being disabled onto a physical obstacle and then one chooses: Sit around feeling sorry for oneself, or soldier on regardless. We're given to believe that wallowing in self-pity is unwholesome (notice that one is never described as "wallowing" in self-esteem) and that tackling the mountain is the healthier choice. Only sometimes, when one has climbed the mountain, what's at the top is raw tempeh.

RIGHT NOW

How do I feel today? How do I feel today compared with how I felt yesterday? How might I feel tomorrow? Am I having a relapse? Am I getting better? If I *am* getting better is it because of the drugs I'm taking, or the nutritional supplements, or my meditations? If I'm feeling *worse,* is it because of the weather, or my diet, or a crisis of faith? Am I having new symptoms? Or are these old symptoms? Are they symptoms I haven't had for awhile, or are they symptoms I've *been* having, but not as intensely as I am having them today? If I decide to pay no attention to MS, will it go away? If I pay MS lots of helpful, caring attention, will it go away?

MS is something you can work with as long as you live. If you want to learn, as many spiritual teachers suggest, that nothing is totally yours to control, here is a subject to practice. Here is a perfectly elegant illustration of the mind gibbering away, trying to find the handle that makes the whole thing work, while the thing itself, MS, goes about its inscrutable, neurochemical business. It isn't like a dog: You can't train it to heel. It isn't like a spouse: You can't negotiate with or divorce it. It isn't like a child: You can't cherish it and then, when it's developed enough, send it on its way.

It might be like a house, though we are admonished not to "dwell" in it. It might be like a swamp, though we are admonished not to "wallow" in it. It certainly has the depth and breadth one associates with geography. We speak of the MS "community," the "road to recovery," the diagnostic "signposts," the "downward path" of the progressive forms. Sounds like a landscape to me. We wander through it, we get lost, we seek direction, we meet one another and travel together.

I want to forgo assigning reasons, anchored in the past, for why I am as I am right now. Not "because I kissed a dog." Not "because I lived in Canada." Not "because I had a virus." I may have done all of those things, or none of them. I want to avoid promising myself that by doing X, Y or Z right now, I can completely influence how I will be in the future. Not "if I have the right amount of faith." Not "if I take so-and-so's expensive nutritional supplement." Not "if I avoid red meat." Not even "if I inject myself regularly." I may do all of those things, or none of them. I am looking for a way to live in the present, to be totally present as I am right now . . . I am right now . . . I am right now . . . .

Imagine that **DEAN KRAMER** *lives in contented seclusion on a farm in rural Pennsylvania with her two beloved terriers and an elderly (human) friend.*

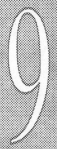

PERSEVERANCE

[EDITOR'S NOTE: *This story is written by Margot Russell about Dr. Richard Radtke.*]

There's a framed image that hangs on the kitchen wall; someplace cold and far away he is holding a penguin, his sky-blue eyes offset by a sea of ice.

The pictures tell a story that words alone cannot. They are the images of a determined man who has traveled the world in a wheelchair.

Dr. Richard Radtke has been to the ends of the earth and even to the bottom of the sea in his chair, researching the dynamics of fish populations and migration as professor of fisheries oceanography at the University of Hawaii at Manoa. He has been hoisted by crane in his wheelchair from a research boat above the Arctic Circle in Norway, lifted by armed guards atop the Great Wall of China and strapped to a bobsled behind a team of dogs in Alaska. No matter what the conditions—perilous, rugged, impossible or otherwise —Dr. Radtke remains undaunted in the face of it all, spurred by the belief that "everyone has a right to fail" on their own.

> I'VE LEARNED TO CONTRIBUTE IN WAYS I DIDN'T KNOW ABOUT BEFORE.
>
> —DR. RICHARD RADTKE

The fact that he has multiple sclerosis and is paralyzed from the neck down lends further proof that the professor defies a simple explanation. When you see a picture of him at the bottom of the ocean in a wheelchair, sporting a scuba tank and mask in the waters off American Samoa, well, you begin to imagine that any limitations we perceive in life may be self-imposed. This is a man who believes that anything is possible, and each day of his life seems a testament to that.

When I first met Dr. Radtke, I had traveled across the entire United States mainland and then six hours over the

Pacific to visit him in Hawaii, hoping to find the answer to a question that had, for years, intrigued me: What is it that motivates people in the face of adversity? Why do some people—their lives profoundly altered by circumstance—march on, sometimes to untold lengths, to succeed? I thought the answer to that question would be quite discernable when I met face to face with it: Dr. Radtke, the epitome of all things brave.

And I wondered how this man in particular—a world-renowned fisheries oceanographer at just forty-seven years old, and the first disabled man to reach Antarctica—could accomplish so much with so little mobility. I had read that Dr. Radtke had seventy publications and numerous scientific meeting presentations to his credit, and that he had traveled to every corner and pocket of the world as a handicapped man collecting samples and thinking deeply about fish. His work has earned him numerous scientific awards, including a nomination to *Who's Who in Science and Technology.*

When I walked into his university office the day after my arrival, it was the quiet that I noticed first: a quiet that emanated from deep concentration, reminiscent of a library, or a church of great renown. Three lab assistants were gathered around a microscope and whenever they or Dr. Radtke spoke, it was always in a whisper.

I noticed the pictures of him, tacked above his desk and gracing the back of a brochure that someone had set out for me. I was most interested in the picture of him dangling high above a research boat in his wheelchair from the scoop of a forklift, and I would come to understand that this was commonplace for him. Radtke has a fondness for heavy machinery, which stems from simple gratitude. When human hands cannot lift him, heavy machinery provides the muscle. Before leaving on a research trip, Radtke calls ahead to the airport, requests a tractor on the tarmac and is lifted to the cargo door of the plane in his wheelchair, while a crowd of awestruck people watches as he leaves.

After a time, he turned to me and apologized for the wait. It was then that I glimpsed the steel-blue eyes, bringing to mind an image of the great wall that lived inside of him—a product, perhaps, of fierce determination and mental might. I sensed that the question I had come to ask had already been answered: His constitution to live life the way he wanted to seemed an inseparable part of him; perhaps it was impossible to extract it and dissect it, forcing upon it the great limitations of words.

While his assistant, Zach, fed him his lunch, we talked about his childhood for awhile: An American childhood it seemed to me, deeply rooted beneath the endless Midwest skies, as he worked on his parents' farm, helping to provide the food that sustained the family of eight. Perhaps his capacity to dream began in those formative years, in those "lazy Indiana summers," when the Radtke brood became easily bored. "Our minds wandered," he said, "and since we were not allowed to watch television, we dreamed of adventures. The West and the cowboys were a popular television topic in the 1960s. Cowboys and soldiers burned in our young minds. Each branch was a gun and every tree an adversary."

I wondered how this experience might be applied to his present life, and so I asked about his trip to Antarctica and how he came to be the first disabled man in that cold and rugged place commonly known as the South Pole.

The South Pole is considered a field of dreams for any marine biologist. Extreme atmospheric conditions provide a unique opportunity to study changes in the environment, important research from both a national and a global perspective. Antarctica is a huge continent, covering 10 percent of Earth's mass and influencing a far greater area in the form of cold air, water currents and migratory seabirds and marine mammals. It's also a storehouse for 70 percent of the world's fresh water.

In the 1990s, a convergence of scientists traveled to Antarctica for study. Geologists conducted research in plate tectonics; glaciologists measured the movement and the layers of ice sheet; and marine biologists like Dr. Radtke studied the local marine food chains. In Antarctica the relatively simple ecosystems are easy for scientists to model, since not much survives in the inhospitable clime of the South Pole. The place is, in effect, a magnet for scientists, but a person has to be quite healthy to study at the bottom of the world, and that's a rule established and enforced by the military. I had heard that

Radtke had been granted special permission to travel to the South Pole, setting a precedent that would later afford other disabled people the same opportunity.

"What was it like," I asked, "to arrive there, to be lifted off the boat in your wheelchair—the first disabled man to breathe the Antarctic air?"

"Well, it was a dream come true, really. I had to go through quite a bit to get there, though. I was already married and living in Hawaii, when my interest to travel and study there was sparked. But while making progress in my research studies, I began to notice an increased problem with my balance and gait—the early signs of multiple sclerosis. Typical of the average person diagnosed with the disease, I was in the prime of my life, just starting a career and planning a family."

Radtke said that within two years of his diagnosis, he was in a wheelchair; within three years, he was considered a legal quadriplegic. He was diagnosed with chronic progressive MS, characterized by a swift and steady progression of the disease and few, if any, periods of remittance. The doctors didn't expect him to live very long.

His wife left him, he says, when the disease became a "bit more than she bargained for." She moved back to the mainland United States with their son. The breakup of his family, combined with uncertainty about whether he would be able to continue his field research from a wheelchair, was more than he could bear.

"I lay on my bed one night, staring at the ceiling, not

able to move, and I just cried. My wife and son were gone, and nothing in my life was certain." On the brink of suicide, Radtke knew he had to find something to believe in again, something beyond the four walls of his room and the ever-present feeling of despair. "Radtke," he said to himself, "you'd better start dreaming." That night he made a pact: "I will either kill myself, or I'm going to live the life I want to live." He lay there late into the night, dreaming of the way his life was going to be, and how he was going to put it all together. He defied the voices that had told him he would never have a career or a family again.

Sometime during that long night, he handpicked the inner qualities he possessed that he'd take along with him: stubbornness and courage, focus and determination. Self-pity and fear were left behind, cast away like the pieces of his past; he was now the cowboy of his childhood dreams.

I imagined Dr. Radtke peering out over the great abyss and, after a moment's reflection, deciding to soar rather than jump. Is it possible, I wondered, to recreate who we are in a moment's time—to become an imagined or altered version of ourselves by merely deciding to do so? I had thought we were all products of the days and years that passed, smoothed over by the rough sands of adversity, now a perfect stone after time had had its way.

But after having made his decision to "live the way I want to live," he woke up the next morning, still unable to move, but decidedly on his way to the South Pole.

He tested the waters by writing a proposal to the National Science Foundation to do some research in Antarctica. At this point, Radtke had been an oceanographer for nine years, and he had been paralyzed for two. Not surprisingly, it wasn't clear to anyone but him that he would be allowed to continue his field research, which was really the essence of his work.

"The proposal got excellent reviews and was accepted," he said, "but they didn't know I was in a wheelchair. To go to Antarctica, you have to pass a physical designed for people in the Navy. As you can see, I'm not capable of passing."

He was granted an exemption, which is possible in certain situations, and allowed to take a less stringent physical test. "Outside of the fact that I can't move, I'm in pretty good health. My heart's good, my blood chemistry looks good and I don't have any other complications." Still, the Navy denied his request to go to Antarctica, stating that Dr. Radtke was a "fire hazard."

"I've never burst into flames in my life!" Radtke mused. "People were taking my dreams away, and I realized then that I could do something to change it. I didn't have to accept it. So, I wrote everybody. I wrote to the president, and I wrote my senator."

Social change is a slow process. Initiated by a single purpose, its seed is carried in the wind until it blossoms in our consciousness. The political climate in Hawaii was perfectly poised in 1987 for any initiative called to better the lives of the disabled. Hawaiian Senator Daniel Inouye was himself disabled, having lost an arm in combat in World War II. The senator took an interest in Radtke's predicament, and met with some key people on Capitol Hill. With Inouye's help, the mechanics of change were put into place. In the end, Dr. Radtke was given full exemption, and he became the first handicapped person ever to reach Antarctica. Never before had a man been wheeled into the facilities at the research station of the National Science Foundation's Polar program. Upon entering the station, Radtke recalled, "Everyone knew who I was. They said they had a file on me a foot thick."

Dr. Radtke soon understood that being granted permission to travel to Antarctica was only half the battle. The physical process of getting there and working there was the other half. Radtke traveled by plane to Argentina, where he picked up a boat and made his way to Palmer, where the research station is located, a five-day journey in itself. "I have to be truthful," he said. "The trip turned into an ordeal. There were certain times when I had to just 'gut it out.'"

His arrival at the bottom of the world would be an introductory lesson in survival. Conditions there are difficult for an able-bodied man, much less a quadriplegic. "Antarctica was not handicapped accessible. They had to use a bosun's chair—a special chair on a boom with a winch and pulley—to lower me off the boat when we arrived."

The eight weeks Radtke spent in Antarctica would test

his determination. Because his wheelchair could not be pushed over the rocky terrain, he was moved around on the lift of a giant motorized snow shovel. Field researchers in Antarctica live and work in direct exposure to the challenging conditions, in what is called the windiest, coldest place on earth. Radtke spent much of his time on a research boat, his wheelchair strapped tightly to the legs of a lab bench, identifying fish as they were hauled up in nets.

It was a lonely time, Radtke says. When not out in the field, he was forced to stay on the first floor of the research facility, because there were no elevators. Isolated from his colleagues, his eight weeks there felt like "solitary confinement." Despite the difficult conditions, the trip was a success. Radtke had proven to himself, and to the gatekeepers of the science world, that he was more than capable; in fact, he was awarded a presidential commendation for his accomplishment. "I realized when I returned home that no one could take my dreams from me," Radtke said. Since then, he has traveled back to Antarctica and made more than fifty research trips to every corner of the world in his wheelchair.

I want to know about the other snapshots, the faded photos lining his office walls: a younger Dr. Radtke in Greenland and Norway, a shot of him in his wheelchair, sporting a scuba mask and oxygen tank at the bottom of the sea. But the stories will wait for another day. I leave to catch a bus back to my hotel, silently questioning the strength of my own dreams.

They come to pick me up in a handicapped-accessible van. I watch as Dr. Radtke's second wife bounds from the driver's seat to fetch me from the curb. Ocean, their seven-year-old daughter is right behind her, curious about me and wanting to play. I show her the stuffed dolphin I have brought her and am instantly corrected: "It's actually a whale," she says.

On the way to their home in the suburbs of Honolulu, Dr. Radtke insists that we stop at an overlook, the perfect place for a snapshot providing a view of the world all around. He is tired and doesn't join us, but his proclivity to show others what he most loves to see is touching.

I realize now that Dr. Radtke whispers to conserve energy. Away from his office—where concentration and solitude have purpose—he still whispers. His voice is quiet, and humbleness emanates from his six-foot four-inch, 200-pound frame. (Radtke played football as a college undergraduate.) Later, I remember him telling me that he couldn't watch football at all after he was diagnosed. It seemed a poignant reminder of what he had lost.

We sit in his living room all afternoon, while the sound of his daughter playing in the yard drifts through the open windows. Clearly, she is the love of his life. His eyes light up when she walks into the room, a testament that his life has carried on—even regenerated—despite the struggle.

I ask him to define his courage. After fumbling for an answer, he says this: "All of our acts, no matter how altruistic, are ultimately done for ourselves, as a way of defining who we are. When I give talks to groups, people come up afterward and thank me for giving such a nice talk. And I want to say, 'No, I want to thank you! You've given me the opportunity to take all of these stories, these things in my life that have caused so much pain, and share them so that they don't hurt anymore.'"

He tells me a moving story about being on Rose Atoll while on a research trip funded by the National Geographic Foundation. He says he spent the first day scuba diving with his two assistants. In the vast warehouse of Radtke's life experiences, perhaps scuba diving is what he treasures most—the wonderful feeling of weightlessness as he sinks to the ocean bottom, his arms and legs buoyant after so many years of paralysis, the cool ocean water teeming with life. The world becomes vivid; his body is comforted; paralysis is a distant memory for a time.

"You get in the water and you feel freedom. And that freedom brings back to you what it was like before, to move on your own. As the day went on, I was getting more and more frustrated remembering how I used to do things. It all came back again. At the end of the day, I was up on the beach watching the sunset, and it was the first day that I just cried. I started to ask myself 'Why am I doing all of this? Why don't I just quit?' And then I realized why. It's not for science or for mankind; it's for me.

"When I was deep down in depression after the first few years in a wheelchair, I did a lot of soul searching. One of the things I realized was that I felt I wasn't any use to the human race. I couldn't move, I couldn't walk, so what use was I going to be to the kid next door? How was I going to contribute to society? But then I started doing some things for nonprofit organizations and I began to realize, my God, I can contribute to the world. I've learned to contribute in ways I didn't know about before."

While his career accomplishments portray a man of great courage and ability, it is Professor Radtke's tireless work with the disabled that others say defines him. With the help of several grants, he has created two nonprofit organizations aimed at getting kids with disabilities interested in science and technology. The Ocean of Potentiality Program, with its camps and Dolphin Interaction Program based in Hawaii, strives to encourage children and youth with disabilities through a hands-on approach to science. Radtke believes that education is a conduit for those with physical or mental disabilities, and that through his example, he can help to show the way. Inspired by his work in Hawaii, Radtke also created the Dream Catchers Project, an organization aimed at getting Alaskan kids with disabilities to envision a better future. In 1999, President Bill Clinton presented Dr. Radtke with an award for his dedication to mentoring children.

I see a picture of Dr. Radtke at camp somewhere, a group of children in front of him, reaching for his lap. His desire for them to see what he sees, to know what he knows, has created an incredible bond.

"When you fly over the tundra and see caribou, it just changes you," he says. "And I don't mean watching it on television. It's when you're there in real life that it really makes a big difference. Once you can show people that the things in life they thought were not possible are possible, then you can change their paradigms. It's like letting the genie out of the bottle."

Jim Skouge, his friend and camp associate, stops by to chat. While discussing Radtke's accomplishments, his eyes fill with tears. "Here's where Richard has played a big role in other people's lives," he says. "When I was a boy, there were a few people who, even if they didn't spend a lot of time with me, I just knew that they were adults who had stopped the clock. They really accepted me and liked me. I think those are the moments when a human being goes through some kind of transformation."

Dr. Radtke and Skouge took some of the kids from the Hawaii camp on a trip to the most "mind-boggling, beautiful spot" in the Hawaiian Islands, believing that experience is the great purveyor of growth. Despite the difficulties in getting there, the trip to Molokai—a remote island that once served as a leper colony—was a success. Indeed, the snapshots reveal a tropical oasis, a gaggle of kids surrounding an old cabin, and for some, it was the first time they had ever left their own back-yards. It was a spot as close to the tundra and the cari-bou as Dr. Radtke could provide. It is this work, I decide—his work with the children that share his own struggles in the world—that brings clarity to his life. The process of giving back provokes a transformation all its own.

We discuss the difficulties of being "waist high in the world," and I begin to sense that part of his motivation to succeed springs from an underlying fear of "the sys-tem." He says he's watched too many people in his situa-tion being "gobbled up" by a system that favors long-term nursing facilities over home health-care aides and attendants.

"What keeps a lot of people in nursing homes is the lack of adequate attendants," he says. "A lot of these people don't have real medical problems that require nursing care. They're just not in a situation where they can afford an attendant. So they go into the system. The crazy thing about it is that it costs the system more to keep them in a nursing home. I've always tried to stay outside of it. I've seen too many people who were gob-bled up by it, and let it run their lives. I just can't see that for myself. I mean, people with handicaps have minds, but society just gives up on them. They put them some place and wait for them to die. I don't want that for myself, or for anybody else."

In part, Radtke has kept ahead of "the system" by thinking outside of the box. After some serious problems with past attendants, he came up with a solution that has so far served him well. He solicits college-age kids from his hometown in Indiana and offers to pay their college tuition and room and board, in exchange for their personal-care services. "You have to set it up so that your attendant is getting some self-worth out of the situation," Radtke says.

Caregivers are often the invisible force in the home of a quadriplegic, who lacks the capability to perform the simple tasks that sustain life. It is the caregivers who provide the key to Dr. Radtke's freedom and independence. They help to funnel the raw potential into solid form. They rouse him from sleep every morning, help to dress him, feed him and get him to work, and deliver him to physical therapy twice a week. His assistants in the lab return phone calls, order the supplies, feed him lunch and transform his mental meanderings into tangible reality. If Radtke's fierce determination is the engine propelling his success, his caregivers are the wings.

When I am ready to leave, I notice a large framed photograph of Dr. Radtke hanging on a wall in the kitchen. He is a young man in the picture, able-bodied, the breeze from a cold and faraway place blowing blonde hair from his face. He has the look of a confident man who is never too far from his dreams. He is holding a penguin in the picture, his razor blue eyes reflecting a strength he'd soon be called upon to muster.

Later, I call him from my hotel. We hadn't talked about his trip to China, when he'd asked the armed guards at the Great Wall to carry him the thirty steps to the top. They not only obliged, but offered to carry him through the Imperial Palace as well. He laughs at the memory. "The translator I'd hired told me that the soldiers were bored, and were having a great time carrying me around. In fact, they all wanted to take turns. I felt like a real king!" The China visit taught him, once more, the lesson he is able to bring to others: "There is always a way."

I ask about the photo of him in his wheelchair at the bottom of the sea. "I don't typically scuba dive in a wheelchair," he says. "We took the picture in American Samoa. I had funds from the National Geographic Foundation to study giant clams on a small atoll called Rose Atoll. I thought it would be kind of fun to have a picture like that, and the wheelchair was in the boat. Of course, a wheelchair in the water is totally worthless. It rusted within a couple of weeks. Saltwater is just horrible on them. But this is a picture of a moment in my life.

"You know, I wake up in the morning, and I might be in pain, but I'm excited. I'm excited to be awake. I'm always looking for a new cliff to jump off. A colleague once asked me 'Rich, why do you do all of this? It's kind of like jumping off a cliff, isn't it?' 'Yes,' I answered, 'but boy is it fun jumping off a cliff. It's a hell of a lot more stimulating. I'm going places that I don't know anything about. I am totally at ease when I know nothing. I love to learn.'"

Soon I am on my way home to the less tropical clime of New England in April, fitting together the pieces of a man I've come to admire. I realize that Dr. Radtke has taught me more about possibility than he has about himself, and that it is not the magnitude of our difficulties that defines us. We are defined, instead, by what we do with them.

Others would argue that it is his tireless search for self-worth that propels him onward, or his determination to "live life the way I have always imagined it." But in the end, the why and the how of it lose their importance. It is the snapshots that bring us inspiration, the faded photographs of a life lived with courage and poise. We see handicapped children sitting on his lap at camp, the setting sun illuminating smiles of tremendous hope. We see him dashing through the impossible snow-laden fields of Alaska behind a team of dogs, and we can envision a future ahead, somewhere beyond the next ridge. He becomes our eyes, way above the world on the Great Wall of China, beneath the bluest water of the ocean's edge.

We are reminded once again, and promised once again, that everything is possible.

DR. RICHARD RADTKE *is a full professor in biological oceanography in the School of Ocean and Earth Sciences and Technology at the University of Hawaii. In just one recent year, Dr. Radtke traveled to Alaska, China, Indonesia, Canada and Greenland to conduct research experiments in oceanography. In his spare time, he has inspired students and adults through special presentations on his work and life and has earned many awards and honors for his volunteer efforts throughout the United States. His other interests include photography, scuba diving, fishing and sailing. Dr. Radtke has also establishd the Sea of Dreams Foundation, which creates programs to assist disabled youth in the United States and abroad. For more information contact* Margot62@aol.com.

MARGOT RUSSELL *has worked as a news broadcaster, a reporter and a television producer. She lives on Cape Cod, Massachusetts, with her family and enjoys sailing, skiing, hiking and traveling in New England and abroad.*

10

SETTING GOALS

Julie Full-Lopez

I was not born brave. I am not that person who will check out a strange sound in the middle of the night—though I've heard a lot of them when illness looms large at 3:00 A.M., and the medicine that I take to fight back this intruder ensures that I will hear the clock chime hourly until daybreak. At least, I reason, if I am awake, parts of my body won't be stolen as I sleep. This is not brave. This is my Olympian stubbornness, a character trait that has taken me to places that insomnia would not let me dream of. This is my life.

Adulthood officially began for me at twenty, and it would soon find me graduating from college and, subsequently, getting married before I turned twenty-two. That was my hope, anyhow—if the double vision would stop. Optic neuritis left me feeling like I had a triple martini for breakfast, lunch and supper; and all the doctors could say was that I should "get my affairs in order." They made it sound like I was rather near death, and I remember wondering what I should wear for such an occasion. All I really had was a wedding gown with a white, puffy, veiled hat.

> MY INSTRUMENTS OF SELF-MEASUREMENT AND ANALYSIS WERE IN NEED OF CHANGE.

After two weeks of a staggering drunken stupor, my vision returned to the standard "one of everything," and I commandingly resumed my wedding plans, rationalizing numb knees and kaleidoscopic four eyes as academic exhaustion. Of course, not every exhausted college student is asked to have a spinal tap and myelogram, and I was nearly certain that my doctors were trying to defraud Blue Cross-Blue Shield, for nothing could be wrong with me. They had the wrong person. I vowed at that moment to prove them wrong. I chose scuba as my therapy, diving to the bottom of the Caribbean on my honeymoon. Sick people never scuba dive.

Well, the honeymoon ended, and by 1982, my doctor suggested that I have a family as soon as possible. A numb kneecap or hand hardly seemed to necessitate offspring, but since I was told I would not pass multiple sclerosis to my child, I thought, what the heck. Matthew was born December 29, 1982, during the total eclipse of a full moon. The pregnancy had been normal, and multiple sclerosis never presented itself during my maternal lactating period. It waited until I had symmetrically stocked the newborn Pampers and color-coded drawers with terry sleepers and onesies. Then it took my arm.

As with many MS attacks that come early in the disease, my numb arm recovered fairly quickly as the intruder relented. Matthew and I bonded for his first four years—years that were punctuated by three to four exacerbations per year. This illness was getting on my nerves. I couldn't understand why the doctors couldn't just stop it.

To sustain hope in myself, I decided to enroll in graduate school, much to the chagrin of my family and doctors—all of whom, preferring caution, thought I needed more rest. I planned to do a master's in English and American literature. When I applied, my undergraduate grade-point average not only got me into school, it also got me a job. So at twenty-five—a married mother with MS—I became a salaried university instructor of expository writing; my own studies would be tuition-free. This turned out to be one of the most exhaustingly, positive experiences of my life, and I was good at it.

What I was not good at, during my first year of graduate school, was walking between classes. I found myself stopping four to five times on outdoor benches between adjacent buildings. This was a fairly inconspicuous thing to do on a campus of fifteen thousand—that is, until it rained or hit subzero temperatures.

I suppose I thought that if I could hide my MS from others, then I could hide it from myself. I simply would not allow myself to be sick, or at least not very sick. But, I began to realize that familiar evasion tactics were not going to work anymore.

Multiple sclerosis is a relentlessly insidious adversary, always looking to come in under the door. Before I was to complete graduate school, my MS resumé would include optic neuritis, double vision, facial and bodily neuropathies, a negative Babinksi's sign in paralyzed feet, neuralgia parasthetica that numbed my legs, and brain MRIs that lit up like Christmas trees. For my new tactic to battle multiple sclerosis, I chose, at the insistence of my friends, counseling. I hated the idea, but it was clear my triple-A, rule-the-world personality needed a nudge. Okay, maybe a life vest. I had to recognize that

MS had gotten to me, not just to my body. My self-confidence was being fueled by my academics, my teaching. But at the end of the day and on into the middle of the night, illness loomed large because it was in me.

In counseling, I was beginning to understand that I was letting fear of the unknown, as well as the actual physical changes MS brought, change the way I saw myself, change the sense of my own identity. Though I feared what multiple sclerosis could do to my body, however, I realized that I was truly afraid of not being emotionally strong enough to meet the physical challenges of the disease. I also had a lot to learn about MS, its treatments (or lack thereof) and the strength in myself that I could no longer calculate in laps, miles or hours at the gym. My instruments of self-measurement and analysis were in need of change. My hands, which were clamped tightly over my eyes for seven years, had kept me from seeing new possibilities for a life with a chronic illness.

A major downside of denial of illness is the denial of response to it by friends and family. Sensing inevitably that nothing is the same in their wives, husbands, daughters, sons or even mommies, friends and family are unable, but desperate, to release an emotional expression of their anguish. In this way MS disables entire families, not just its reluctant hosts.

I found that children may feel shut out the most: first, because they are afraid when mommy is sick, and also, because they simply lack the vocabulary to talk about what will turn into upset stomachs, headaches, lost blankies and sick stuffed animals. My son Matt had many of these childhood infirmities, some at day care where abandonment seemed certain, and other times at soccer and baseball games, when it was too hot for me to watch from the stands with other parents. Heat and MS don't mix, but on the longest, hottest, most perfect summer's day, that line drive to deep left field ends up feeling more like a lost blankie.

I knew my occasional absence from the baseball diamond, soccer field, city parade, picnic, swimming pool or any other outdoor event would not be looked upon favorably by my family. My limitation, however, was too new for them to fully understand. St. Louis summer heat is especially unforgiving to one with MS. I found myself going to the grocery store by 7:00 A.M., before the heat of the day. I was left feeling rather like an astronaut forced to retreat to the dark side of the moon before the sun heats up the lunar surface.

My fellow astronauts, my son and husband, though tolerant of my choice to study indoors rather than explore moon craters with them, probably felt abandoned at times—just as I felt abandoned by my former self. This kind of thing can go by day to day, nearly unnoticed; then at other times, the searing wounds created by harsh words of misunderstanding can isolate family members from each other—sometimes forever.

As a graduate student with loads of homework and nearly as much grading of papers to do, I had to spend much of my time sitting, which was fortunate for me. Academic work also freed me from dwelling too much on just how hard it was on my family for me to have MS, and it gave me a productive way to cope with fatigue, the worst "f" word imaginable to most people who have multiple sclerosis. MS fatigue can make everyday personal-care activities—showering, dressing, blow-drying—exhausting tasks. Grooming my son meant performing these activities twice—along with packing lunches, retrieving runaway pets, carpooling and racing to my own classes with a twenty-five-pound *Riverside Shakespeare* in hand. That book was heavy enough to prepare me for an Olympic shot-put competition. I wonder if this is what the Bard had in mind when he said, "Sweet are the uses of adversity."

As a mother to a five-year-old, wife, student, teacher and doer of all things not necessarily necessary, I learned that I was going to have to learn how to manage my time more efficiently, capitalizing on peak energy periods for the most demanding tasks and responsibilities. This meant that I would have to book classes more in the first part of the day and sit and grade as the day progressed. I would also have to learn to eat better—

French roast coffee is not a food group. I needed more energy-sustaining, slow-burning foods.

Eating properly is good in theory, but I found it hard to do within a hectic 8:00 A.M. to 5:00 P.M. schedule that did not relent just because I had arrived home from work and school. In fact, it rather seemed like the day was beginning anew with supper, dishes and homework.

As my comprehensive exams grew nearer, I could see the light at the end of the graduate school tunnel. I studied all day, then all night, except for Friday evening when my family would go out to dinner. I had my fingers crossed that at graduation I would be able to walk independently across the stage; but my on-again, off-again exacerbations kept me in constant doubt. If I had needed a cane or elbow to lean on, it wouldn't have made my honor any less. But I had worked hard to reach my goal, and I wanted it all to myself. I did not want to share any of my glory with my disease, for I felt it did not deserve it.

I passed my exams, all seventy-two pages of them. Garbed in a sexy, yet "I am successful" dress with medium heels and matching purse, along with the "royal robes," mortarboard, and master sash, I walked—no, floated—across the stage. I certainly showed my MS who was in charge that day in 1987, as it deferred its power over me.

I was offered a full-time teaching position at the university I had attended. I needed this: I needed something that I was good at, something I could do even when my limbs were not being totally cooperative. After my divorce three years later, my wounds of insecurity felt ripped wide open. If I learned anything in college, it was that there is always more to learn, and life was going to have such an array of disappointments and victories for me that I could not have fathomed them.

The first time divorce had ever entered my mind came five or six years before my husband and I separated, about the time I was starting grad school. I hadn't anticipated that college would teach me so much, and not just about academics: I learned about myself, about that person who was trying to get out, get free, who just for once wanted to do what was not sensible, cautious or doctor "prescribed" and mother "approved."

I was also looking for that person I had only met in passing, in the library, at a party, in the classroom. She was that person who looked back at me every morning when I greeted her with hot coffee and reluctant sleepy eyes. It turned out that she was me in the mirror, and I realized that I forgot to get to know her, for she was juggling a family, school, a career. She was also spending half her time hiding from a disease that would never go away; the other half she spent hiding from the world when MS left her feeling awkward, dependent, maybe even ugly.

I had grown distant from my husband, in part because I was growing in ways I could never have anticipated while in college. I also grew distant as I began to feel more like a liability and not a lover, not a life partner. It was then that I took my life back. I owed it to those eyes that unfailingly looked back at me every morning, beckoning me to do the right thing, not my family's thing, or my in-law's thing or even that wife thing, but *my* thing.

For two years after my divorce, I remained in remission, a condition I had never known during my entire adult life. My neurologist attributed it to the lower stress levels in my life, relief from the stress of marital unrest. I did not really care what caused the prolonged remission, but I enjoyed life in ways I had never dared.

My son and I, along with a couple of my girlfriends, went to a Colorado dude ranch. Cowboy hats, spurs and all, we rode every day for a week, up and down mountains along the Continental Divide. Weak knees, nothin'! My palomino, Tennessee, took me to heights I could never have climbed on my own. This was a good, physical activity that my son and I both could do, and the mountain temperature suited me fine. We would repeat this adventure several more times throughout my son's teenage years. Dangerous? Probably, but it was so empowering to be able to do "regular stuff" with my son. Okay, maybe the Continental Divide isn't exactly "regular;" but it made memories to last a lifetime, memories to get me through the hard times that can come with multiple sclerosis. I have learned to book exciting vacations whenever I come out of remission, for there has to be something "wonderful" to look forward to, particularly when MS leaves me feeling, at times, as though life may never be the same again.

When I was not accepted into the trials for a new MS drug that was being tested, I stepped out of my silence and began to educate myself about the politics of drug approval in the United States. Only twenty thousand MS patients were eligible for the trials, and I was told I would have to wait. First, I wrote to the appropriate agencies in Washington, D.C., to protest drug shortages and limited accessibility, as I assumed those constituted the problem. I found out that the Food and Drug Administration (FDA) has no control over individual pharmaceutical companies or how, when or how much medicine they produce. It takes up to fifteen years to approve new drugs for consumers; and once approved, liability and production costs can limit the initial amounts made available. As a result, medical "ethicists" devise drug accessibility lotteries—otherwise known as hope.

Snowballs do tend to grow as they roll down mountains, and I personally wanted to drop an avalanche on MS. I accepted a role as spokesperson for the St. Louis

Gateway Area Chapter of the National Multiple Sclerosis Society (NMSS), not quite sure what I was to speak about. I learned, however, that if I educated myself on the medical issues surrounding MS and its treatments, and spoke sincerely and from the heart, I really couldn't go wrong. From 1993 to 1994, as I waited for my "lucky number" to be called, I began a personal campaign of MS patient education. While letters arrived from the executive secretariat of the FDA in Washington, D.C., I spoke at hospitals and universities, and I began taping television shows about disabilities for cable and prime-time "Health Beat" reports by some of the local stations. I never considered myself doing such things; I did them in the hope of helping people with MS, as well as their families and friends.

My political training was advanced by a group called Pharmaceutical Researchers and Manufacturers of America, for whom I worked in Washington on a number of occasions in 1995 and 1996. A small delegation of people with, or representing people with, various diseases testified before Congress on health-care reform bills, ones that directly or indirectly would affect our lives. Our work finally paid off as the Kennedy-Kassebaum bill was passed by Congress. This bill allows for the "portability" of insurance, meaning that a history of health insurance coverage at one job guarantees coverage, without exceptions, at a new job. People with disabilities are often hesitant to change jobs for fear of losing insurance coverage at the next. My work in Washington was empowering, but the excitement was only beginning in my life.

I had started interferon treatment, and surprisingly, the next knock on my door came from the very company that manufactures my medicine. It had obtained my name from the St. Louis NMSS chapter, for which I had been so active. Out of the blue, I was asked to go to London, England, with a delegation of five MS patients who were among the first to embrace interferon therapy. Before I could leave that summer to fly to London, I was asked to be in the 1996 Summer Olympics. My event would be the one-kilometer torch run through St. Louis.

I proudly told everyone I knew. After all I had endured with this disease, through physical therapy, noodle knees, canes, limping and outright tantrums, I must have elevated my event to the level of the heptathalon in all of our minds.

My Olympic entourage, complete with motorcycle police troopers, led me through the St. Louis streets. People lined both sides of the highway to get a glimpse of this Olympian with a fiery gold torch longer than a baseball bat. I do not think the crowd was aware that I had had multiple sclerosis for sixteen years by that point, and I'll bet they did not know that I was afraid of tripping and falling. The United Way people may have known; they had nominated me a "Community Hero" for all of my volunteer work. I was one of ten thousand people needed to carry the Olympic flame across the country, and at that moment, I was as proud as I had ever been. This was my personal dose of hope to 350,000 Americans with multiple sclerosis. I would soon find, however, that there still was not enough medicine to go around.

After my Olympic torch was snuffed out, I continued to bask in the public spotlight, thanks to a tenacious Associated Press photographer who sent my moment of Olympic glory around the world. In England, we were treated like celebrities (royalty, if you will) and treated to amenities such as stretch BMWs, chauffeurs, theatre, fine hotels, television, newspapers and call-in radio shows during which MS patients could ask us about the newest therapy. Rumor had it that the treatment was far worse than the disease, and patients were eager to see what they thought would be "the face of death" from MS therapy. What they received was one of the first clinical-trial patients, an engineer, an oncology nurse, an active housewife and me, an "Olympian."

As word spread, I suppose, that we weren't dead, we were escorted through London: Prince Charles's flat, Buckingham Palace, the Palladium Theatre. We hung out with British MS patients, all eager to hear our stories, to learn about our side effects. I reported that the biggest side effect was on my wallet, at $10,000 per year—and the treatment I was using was not even a cure. All but one of the British patients I met said they could not get medicine to slow the progression of their MS.

As of May 2000, Reuters has reported an MS popula-
tion of 85,000 in the United Kingdom, with only 3 percent getting therapy. The United Kingdom's universal
medical care system was actually considering ending the
expensive treatments altogether. And I had been angry
because I had to "wait my turn" for MS medicine! What
if I lived in a country that could decide for me how I may
or may not be treated when ill or disabled? I said my
good-byes to the British that summer, but we promised
each other that we would meet again. I left counting my
blessings, as delayed as they sometimes seem to be.

When my MS came on with a vengeance in 1998, I
remember altering my original deal with God. This time, a
permanent cane-assisted limp would be okay—not great,
but okay. I just wanted this attack to stop moving, claim-
ing my body and deadening me to the bone. My neurologist seemed extra thoughtful during this time, sometimes
phoning on Saturday to see how I was doing. She kept
reminding me that I had a triple-A personality, but that I
wasn't able to fix this, much less deal with it. She was
right. Steroids and an elevated dose of interferon were to
be my short-term and long-term goals, respectively.

I remained on the cane for quite a few weeks, but was
finally able to let it go, satisfied with a heavy limp.
Multiple sclerosis attacks with exponential force, yet

retreats fractionally and over a long period of time. I've never been particularly patient, but 1998 changed me. I have never appreciated doing laundry, carpooling or even mopping the floor as much as I do today. I clearly remember when these tasks were "physical luxuries," and today, I am glad to be strong enough to enjoy them. I still complain, of course, but I do have a reputation to uphold. I am a mom.

I hope to publish my own book soon, and to go back to London with it to tell my British friends that I have not forgotten them. I hope my efforts there will help them to have greater access, soon, to new multiple sclerosis therapies. I truly believe that no one, anywhere, should be denied therapies that can slow the progression of this disease, the greatest crippler of young adults aged twenty to forty.

JULIE FULL-LOPEZ *is a single parent and a twenty-year veteran of MS. She is also a writing instructor at Southern Illinois University at Edwardsville, Illinois, teaching additional general education and medical law and ethics classes at Sanford-Brown College. Julie is a volunteer and spokesperson for the St. Louis Gateway Area Chapter of the National Multiple Sclerosis Society. She is a past recipient of the NMSS Individual Achievement of the Year Award. Julie continues to be an activist for medical reform in the United Kingdom.*

11

REMEMBERING DREAMS

Margot Russell

I paused for a moment to catch my breath and readjust my gear. We had already climbed several hundred feet up the mountain, and I was slowly becoming ill from the altitude. I had fallen behind my group by stopping to rest, fighting off the dizziness and physical fatigue.

Below me, the gentle Urubamba River curved gracefully along the valley in the Andes Mountains of Peru. It had been just three hours since jumping off the rustic train from Cuzco with the others, literally in the middle of nowhere, to begin our hike along the ancient Inca Trail to Machu Picchu. Now, I was several thousand feet up the mountain and had miles to go before we stopped for the night. I was battling fatigue, altitude sickness and my own uncertainty that I would make it to the top.

For almost half my life, I had wanted to travel to Machu Picchu. I think I stumbled upon a picture of it in my younger years, and it became an icon of what the endless world had to offer. It seemed a place of mystery and hidden adventure, a place that ordinary travel could not take you.

> I WAS ALSO
> A STRONG WIND OF
> POTENTIAL AND BEAUTY,
> BLOWING QUIETLY AWAY
> . . . FROM THE LAND OF
> COULDN'T BE.

The world is such a magnificent place; its pockets full of exotic coins and drawers of foreign fabric. I imagine that we'd all like to collect a trinket or two from the corner of everywhere and dangle them like charms from a bracelet.

We dream of the places we will go; we dream of the things we can do. We are dancing on a slow boat down the Nile. We are taking tea with the Queen, having remembered our gloves. We bring those dreams out like an old party dress from time to time, and try them on for size. We wonder if they still fit.

Years before I finally got there, my Machu Picchu dream resurfaced with a surprising reverie. My father was traveling around the world, and I imagined I could meet him if he stopped there.

It was an idea whose time had not come. I was the mother of three little girls, and my husband and I were laying bricks. We had only the station wagon, not the white picket fence or a family dog. Dreams of travel were in the file marked "extravagant."

I had been taught that travel was something you earned. It's a retirement gift you give to yourself, or something you do in the Navy. For us ordinary folk, far away from the fur-clad women on the deck of the *Titanic,* travel was extraordinary.

But when my father returned from his adventure two years later—freshly tanned, knapsack full of maps and trinkets—I began to see travel as an ordinary membrane that I could pass through. He had often lived in a tent and eaten by the campfire with other adventurers who were hoping to see a different sky. He had forsaken fancy hotels and expensive restaurants in lieu of the road less traveled. My vagabond thoughts were changed forever; anyone could be a Christopher Columbus.

My life had begun to change, too, and there was now open space to consider. My future stood before me like a vast, endless plain. I was divorced and struggling to provide a life for my children. I was a madwoman, running to my job as a radio news reporter, and then running to daycare afterward. I would gather my children by the scruffs of their necks and plunk them down in the kitchen, where yesterday's dishes and last month's bills crowded our thoughts and the countertops.

It wasn't until I was diagnosed with multiple sclerosis that I began to take deep breaths and tear down the landscape that I had created unknowingly.

And everything would change.

My guide, Lios, a short Peruvian about twenty-four years old, stayed behind with me as our group of more experienced hikers raced ahead. I was taking such quick deep breaths that my abdominal muscles ached; it became obvious that I was struggling with the climb. I had never been so thirsty in my life, and I drank from my canteen as if it contained the last few drops of water in Peru.

Lios seemed troubled by my lack of physical stamina, and I wondered if I should explain. I had obviously overestimated my strength. We paused at a thatched hut for a rest, as the golden sun rose high above the mountaintops. I have traveled a long way in my life to be here, I decided. There was no other choice but to forge ahead.

An hour and a half later, the world took on a brighter hue. I began to adjust to the altitude: My breathing slowed, the dizziness disappeared and I knew that I would make it the rest of the way.

I left my job as a reporter shortly after my diagnosis, and spent the next year or so staring out of the picture window in the kitchen. There was nowhere to go. I couldn't appreciate the silence in my life, because it felt like emptiness.

It was the only time that I can remember in my life when I wasn't striving for control. Instead of packing the picnic lunch, I was merely the cloud above, restless and wandering in the wind. I stopped visiting friends. I turned down invitations. My existence hinged solely on my illness.

I spent my days fighting with insurance companies and poring over medical journals. Vitamin bottles reproduced in my cupboards. I tried yoga and meditation, but my heart wasn't there. In between gulps of brown rice and barley, I watched soap operas and game shows and decided not to ponder my existence anymore.

I view that period of my life now as a great slowing of the engines. Racing down the track full steam, the view of the lilacs and distant smokestacks were obscured by headlong flight; the point of convergence was always up ahead. It was a time of silent, indulgent sobriety, but it served to refocus my view. I was back to kitchen work: reorganizing the pots and pans, scrubbing the floors and the walls of a tired soul. I had to begin again, a most long and painstaking task.

As I made my way, planting small seeds in an empty garden, I found delight in simple things—shuffling through a forest of tall pines, painting the wall in the living room the most lively color of pumpkin. I revisited old dreams for a time and decided I would travel. I wanted to trek to a place of ancient origin, where clarity was bequeathed from the mountaintops, and where the motion of my feet would bring me to a better view.

We arrived at sunset at a large complex high up in the mountains that housed hundreds of hikers on their way to the mysterious land of Machu Picchu. The rest of my group went to explore the area where our tents were set up, but I dropped onto a stone terrace, barely able to move. I had never been so tired or dirty in my life. I sat alone for hours, listening to the voices of strangers. I missed my family and wondered why I had dragged myself to the top of the world like this.

Thoughts of the day drifted through my mind. I recalled the 200-foot waterfall we had passed in the morning, and the brook in the rain forest where we had stopped to eat our lunch. We had hiked past ancient ruins and temples left unscathed by time. I was, I thought, privileged to experience such grandeur.

At dinner, made by our porters late in the evening, I declined all but the soup. I was physically and mentally exhausted, but somehow I reveled in my new persona: explorer, wanderer, dirty mother high up in the mountains donning dusty hiking boots. It occurred to me that just a year before, I had lain in a hospital bed in Boston for treatment of a nasty MS episode. Today, I felt like Indiana Jones.

After a cup of tea made from coca leaves and boiling water, we climbed a mile farther up the mountain to our tents. I was the only single person in my group, so I had a tent to myself, pitched right next door to a small shack inhabited by a Quechua Indian woman. The Quechua, descendants of the Incas, still live a very primitive life farming in the mountains of the Andes.

Built sometime around 1400 A.D., Machu Picchu was presumably a spiritual center for the Incas, who inhabited a large section of South America a thousand years after the death of Christ. The Incas were master builders and masons, incredible engineers and stout environmentalists. They sought to harmonize the work of humans with the work of nature. They worshipped the water, the land and the sun, as they did their gods, and they built temples of thanks in places of incredible beauty. Machu Picchu had been built high up in the mountains, at over eight thousand feet—a difficult place to reach. The Spanish never discovered it, even after they had conquered the Incas.

We had planned to awaken for breakfast at 3:00 in the morning, and then begin the final leg to Machu Picchu. I lay there, alone in my tent, taking stock of my physical condition. The familiar numbness and tingling in my arms, a common symptom of MS, had started hours earlier. My legs ached and I was short of breath, yet I felt so alive. I had an unknown source of energy and strength surging through my veins and welling up into my heart like a fountain.

I tried to sleep, but a rooster, two donkeys and the

glorious spirit of the unknown kept me up most of the night. Lios rattled my tent at 3:00 A.M. with a cup of coca tea. We would wind our way up to Machu Picchu now . . . in the dark. I felt strangely energized and ready for the day.

When you've been a mother for a number of years, it's hard to slip away to Peru unnoticed. Your children wonder who will pick up the balled socks under their beds; they worry that next you'll be off to the Congo. Not having set a precedent for hiking alone in the mountains, I had a few questions to answer—but most everyone supported my dream.

At the very heart of humanity, I think, lies a divine pool of possibility. All that we create is simply borrowed from there. We recognize the dreams of others as our own. And so I went away, metaphorically taking the trip down the Amazon for my mother, or the ride on Space Mountain for my children. My knapsack was full of the little dreams of others.

My adventure to Peru would become the standard of my dreams. Having left as a blank slate, I gathered the wide, toothless smiles of the natives, collected long, endless days from the Sacred Valley and saved the droplets of my toil along the ancient trail. I gathered these things, as if they were a harvest, and lived my life abundantly.

I tiptoed along the darkened path like an Indian, listening for the sounds of the wild, carefully planting one foot in front of the other. I urged Lios to go ahead with the group, as I had found my own pace and was reveling in a quiet space and the solitude of thought.

Traveling alone is a solitary flight, where one experiences her own definition of courage. Alone, the trip is not colored by a companion's needs or wishes. You carry your own baggage. You sing your own song. You are free to define the world with your very own words.

And so, on this morning, making my way to this ancient Incan temple in the sky, I began the long task of redefining myself: not as a courageous MS victim, battling the demons with swords and hiking boots, but rather as a capable woman, who could look up the mountain and walk to the top.

Below me, somewhere in another place, my life awaited. My children waited for my return—with safe and caring people in our house by the sea. My disease waited in dark empty rooms for slivers of light to unmask it. And still, the questions that had haunted me whispered softly in my sleep: Will I always walk? Will I hold my daughter's hand as she walks down the aisle? Will anybody want me now?

The sun began to rise slowly, illuminating the once dark shadows of majestic mountaintops, mist rising from the peaks like white puffs of heaven floating home. Ahead of me . . . a set of Incan steps shooting straight up to the sky—the last and hardest stretch. If I can climb just two at a time—if I can take the next step. . . .

Beyond the steep staircase stood a temple bestowing a

glorious view of Machu Picchu nestled in a mountain far below. Other hikers stood silently about: speechless, breathless at the sight. Tall, majestic mountains encircled the ruins, the thin air making it appear that you could touch a peak, wrap it up and take it home.

Seeing that no one had begun to walk the final leg of the trail, I sped ahead to enjoy it alone. I delighted in the solitude, for even the silence seemed to reverberate from the mountaintops, the absence of sound a sound in itself. Light radiated from a clear blue sky, bouncing off the leaves and making patterns on the grass. And always below me I could see the ancient peaks of Machu Picchu jutting boldly toward the sky. They seemed to know that I was coming and welcomed me there.

I arrived with staggering steps and climbed upon an old stone farming terrace that offered a plot of grass and a magnificent view of the world below. Warm tears found their way from my eyes as I whispered, "I am here, I am here!"

And I, at that moment, the sum of all the things I had ever been, found a world inside of me of all the things I might become.

No longer was I just a human being with imperfections and struggles, or a single woman with MS. I was also a strong wind of potential and beauty, blowing quietly away . . . from the Land of Couldn't Be.

Margot Russell *has worked as a news broadcaster, a reporter and a television producer. She lives on Cape Cod, Massachusetts, with her family and enjoys sailing, skiing, hiking and traveling in New England and abroad. Margot collected and edited the stories for this book. She has also been named the executive director of the Sea of Dreams Foundation, created by Dr. Richard Radtke to improve the lives of the disabled both in the U.S. and abroad. She works part time as a reporter for National Public Radio in Falmouth, Massachusetts.*

12

FACING LOSS

Richard Palmer

During my career as a lawyer, I had taken the depositions of dozens of neurologists, though I had never been the patient of one. When my private law practice began in 1985, I defended big drug companies who had been sued: The plaintiffs claimed the pharmaceuticals they ingested had caused unreasonable side effects. My first set of cases involved the DPT vaccine, given to almost every baby in the United States to prevent diphtheria, tetanus and whooping cough. In the cases I was involved in, the babies experienced some "neurological symptoms" shortly after receiving the shot. Their families would file suit and the depositions of the neurologists would begin.

I loved questioning neurologists and trying to find holes in their logic, discovering the facts that they had either neglected or ignored. Arguing with doctors over MRI findings was especially satisfying. I'd often hire a neuroradiologist to feed me tough practice questions before we went to trial. Then I would unload the newly gleaned information on some unsuspecting pediatric neurologist who had probably had a tough day already. I couldn't have known that someday I'd become vastly familiar with the world of neurology, or that an MRI would be the catalyst that would forever change my life.

> IT'S FRIGHTENING
> HOW MUCH OF
> MY SELF-WORTH WAS
> TIED UP IN
> MY JOB.

Becoming a lawyer was not just a means to an end for me; it was the great purveyor of my growth. It marked the first time in my history that I felt inclined to peer inside my own head and observe the inner workings of my mind. I had hardly given my own intelligence a second thought while I was growing up; I had never been very academically motivated in high school. I avoided every class I could and scored average to poor in the classes I did complete. I just wanted to be out of school, get a job and be on my own. I spent most of my spare time during high school working for a fast-food restaurant and driving a Zamboni ice machine at the local skating rink.

It wasn't until I graduated from high school and married my high school sweetheart that I began to look further down the road: past the worn fences of my own hometown, beyond the edges of my own limitations. My wife and I moved to Chicago and began working our way through undergraduate school while I continued to work full-time. After spending two years bending metal tubes between the hours of midnight and 7 A.M. for a local factory that made earth-moving equipment, I finally started appreciating my studies. It seemed the more I used my brain, the faster I thought, and the more ideas I came up with. I was continually amazed by my own capacity to learn. I never felt "smart" until the day I graduated college with a magna cum laude degree in economics. Suddenly, my brain was alive and it had a quickening appetite for knowledge.

I gladly gave up all forms of employment during law school and used my mind at least eighteen hours a day to read, to memorize, to analyze and to think. I left the follies of my younger years behind: the Zamboni ice machine and metal tubes were replaced by common law and torts.

When law school ended, I accepted a job with the federal government as a law clerk to a federal district court judge. For two years, I watched skilled trial attorneys try cases, and I absorbed myself in researching and writing court opinions.

I had watched my own metamorphosis with an air of quiet restraint, but soon I felt compelled to apply myself with confidence to the working world. After I left the judicial clerkship, I took a job as an associate attorney at a big law firm. I spent a lot of time defending big corporations that had been sued because of injuries caused by their products. I worked long hours in a well-pressed suit, pulling the strings of success. I'd arrive home to my wife and our one-year-old son after a long day of work, as if returning home to the castle after a day of slaying dragons with the boys.

With somewhat naïve enthusiasm, I began to compose that long list of expectations for my life, including good fortune, a happy marriage and years of good health. I wasn't prepared for the painful failure of my marriage; when walking in the door to silence required a talent for denial that I did not possess. I did what I did best instead: I worked.

Weekends became another part of the work week. Although my mind still had an insatiable desire to learn, my emotions were dulled and denied. I was lonely; but at least, I consoled myself, I was learning.

The period of self-imposed isolation ended when I met

Connie in 1989. Her dark brown eyes seemed to look deeply inside my soul. Emotions that I had pushed aside suddenly came alive again. She awakened a part of me that I had hidden away since high school. We laughed and we hugged; we rode bikes and walked on the beach. I proposed to her on a warm day in August at our local zoo. We gathered a few of our close friends and family members and married on May 26, 1990.

There are years that ask questions and years that answer, and the days and months after meeting Connie seemed a reply to my silent pleadings for fulfillment. We wanted to make up for lost time in our lives and have a taste of everything the world had to offer. We both became certified scuba divers and once spent a day diving with sharks. We bungee jumped and learned to ski. We decided to buy a boat, and then a plane, and while on one of our weekends away, we sat with a native Indian guide watching the sunrise over rock canyons near the Hopi Indian Reservation in Arizona.

We also developed a passion for our garden and all things green. We landscaped and planted our backyard with enthusiasm, the plants representing, I suppose, the miracle of growth. Our lives and our gardens were blooming with possibility.

I cried tears of joy at Kevin's birth two years after our marriage; I felt complete. My deep need for knowledge and work seemed to be balanced by enjoyment of family and inner growth.

But life is what happens when you're busy making other plans. The weekend before Thanksgiving 1997, I woke up feeling as though I were coming down with a head cold. The only thing missing from my cold was cold symptoms. Although I went to work Monday and Tuesday, I felt tired and dizzy; my words came out slurred, and I soon discovered I couldn't write. I wasn't aware of the problems with my memory at first, because I was much more fascinated with my slurred speech, double vision, imbalance and weakness in my right hand. I took off Wednesday and spent most of the Thanksgiving weekend close to my bed.

A few days later, while running errands, my vision doubled and I had to pull over. I made it home by driving on side streets and covering one eye with my hand.

I called my internist the next morning and went in for my first neurological exam. The doctor assured me that I probably had an inner ear infection, but he reluctantly scheduled me for an MRI.

My internist called me Friday evening with the "results" of my MRI. I say "results" loosely, because I soon learned that *nothing* in neurology would ever be communicated as a "result." Instead, I was told that some neuroradiologist had an "impression" that my MRI was "compatible with a demyelinating process." In my doctor's opinion, the "lesions may represent an initial presentation of MS." He had already made an appointment for me with a neurologist for Monday.

I really didn't know anything about MS. What bothered me most was the thought of having "lesions" in my brain. I had come to value my intelligence, to depend on it, and having lesions, it seemed to me, was like being diagnosed with brain cancer. I hit the books and the Internet to learn all I could about MS and the dreaded lesions before Monday morning.

I found myself admitted to the hospital on Monday, after my second neurological exam. Despite a slew of tests, I still did not get an MS diagnosis. The label I received was "post-viral demyelinating syndrome." The doctor said it might never happen again and that I'd probably feel "out of it" for a while, so when I went to our firm's Christmas party and found I could barely function or speak, I left early without thinking much about it. I still had symptoms, but they seemed to be improving every day.

By January, my work had returned to its normal pace; depositions, hearings and settlement conferences all suddenly appeared on my calendar. My first clue that all was not well came when I tried to settle a case on the phone with the opposing attorney. I outlined with her the details of our settlement proposal, responded to her demands and then immediately called my client for approval. The three-minute delay between calls was too long. By the time I talked to my client, I could not remember what I had discussed minutes earlier. My notes made no sense. I called back the opposing attorney, trying to figure out what we had discussed. By the end of the day, I thought the case had been settled, but I couldn't remember the terms. I slept very little that night.

In less than two months, my nineteen years of schooling seemed to evaporate. I started journaling everything I did or said throughout the day. I also wrote down all of the abnormal things that were happening to me. Some of the earlier symptoms had improved, like balance and vision, but I realized that my brain was not working like it had. My memory was failing me, and I became nervous talking to people. I could see the words on a page, but I could not read them. My thinking had slowed, and taking notes didn't seem to prevent the confusion.

I was not at all happy that my doctor was blaming my symptoms on stress. I had lived through many stressful events over the years, and I had never experienced cognitive problems. I decided not to believe the neurologist, and assumed he was just having a bad day. Instead, I made an appointment with my internist. Certainly, my doctor of fifteen years would get to the bottom of these problems and give me some relief.

My internist, however, felt certain that I had MS. He explained that it would probably worsen over time, and that I was suffering from a psychological reaction to its onset. He prescribed Prozac and told me to skip the psychiatrist.

Driving home from the appointment, I found myself in a daze and drove twenty miles past my house. I "woke up" not at all sure where I was, or how to get home. I called my wife from a phone booth, and she immediately came to retrieve me.

I became a psychiatry patient on January 16, 1998. The doctor had a nice office in a high-rise in downtown Chicago. I sat in the waiting room, listening to relaxing music and reading. The doctor opened the door, waved me in to his couch and said, "Good morning." Then he was silent.

I quickly mustered all of my nineteen years of education, three years of law school, two years of judicial clerkships and nearly fifteen years of litigation practice. I tried to convince the doctor that I was not crazy—not even "stressed." I thought I could convince him within an hour that this whole appointment was a mistake, and that my neurologist just needed to run some more tests. As the doctor listened, he scribbled some notes.

At the end of our session, he gave me the name of a neuropsychologist who could arrange a battery of neuropsychological tests. He claimed that he wanted a "baseline" of my neurological functioning. I was skeptical, but I made the appointment anyway; talking to him had actually made me feel better.

My only experiences with a neuropsychologist had been in a courtroom. During a trial, neuropsychologists are often called upon to determine if someone is competent to stand trial. When I showed up at my appointment a week later, I expected to find a dark room with men in white coats. I was wrong again. The doctor greeted me warmly, took me into his office and quietly shut the door. His southern accent was refreshing, after spending most of the past two months dealing with doctors who talked too fast. Without taking any notes, he asked me why I was there. I started from the beginning: "I thought I was coming down with a head cold. . . ."

Eight hours later, I felt as if I were brain dead. The string of tests administered to me were the hardest tests I'd ever taken—harder than all of the LSATs, SATs and ACTs combined. It seemed that every aspect of my brain was explored. I could barely drive home.

I didn't know whether I wanted the results of the tests to be normal or abnormal. I thought that a normal result would mean I was crazy, and an abnormal result would mean I was brain damaged—not a wealth of good choices. When I returned to the psychiatrist's office two weeks later, he said I wasn't crazy. He explained that it had been a very stressful couple of months, and that stress likely affected my memory and some of my cognitive functioning. He complimented me on my coping skills and the strong support at home. He felt that the stress would lessen over time, after a clear diagnosis was reached.

He then read parts of the report to me: "Moderately severe memory impairment. . . . Moderately slowed mental and response speed. . . . Difficulty with nonverbal perceptual skills. . . . Mild word retrieval difficulty. . . . The significance of these findings is that they represent substantial cognitive impairment in memory and mental speed, which will affect his job performance and every-day life adjustment."

I was speechless. I felt terrible, as if someone had taken a knife, opened up my skull and destroyed large portions of my brain. If I hadn't needed a psychiatrist when I met this man, I certainly needed one now. I made an appointment to return in one week.

A litigator's job at a large law firm is defined by stress. I had grown accustomed to having very little sleep, making important deadlines and working on several projects at once. Now, my doctors were advising me to do just the opposite: avoid stress, get plenty of rest, slow down, avoid deadlines and try to work on only one project at a time. I cancelled as many court hearings and depositions as I could.

It wasn't long before I became stressed out anyway. I couldn't sleep. The deadlines kept looming—and it felt as if I were drowning at work. I didn't tell anyone. My colleagues, and even my secretary, thought I had a bad ear infection. In March, I tried to take a deposition. What a mistake.

Reassured that my speech, right hand and balance were all back to normal, I flew to Florida, rented a car and drove to a golf club to take a deposition from a retired distributor for a medical device company. I had spent several hours getting organized and writing out questions. As depositions go, this one should have been easy. The witness was sworn—and suddenly my mind went blank. The stress had caused my speech to slur, and then my right hand became weak. My memory left me entirely—though I continued to read the questions on my list as the court reporter typed the witness's answers. I was done in less than an hour, and I walked outside to try to figure out what had happened. One of the other attorneys told me that I looked ill, and I agreed; I told him it was a cold I had caught the night before. I jumped in the car and headed for the airport. After missing several exits and stopping to ask for directions twice, I finally found the airport and crawled on the last flight back to Chicago. That would be the last deposition of my career.

I know a lot of lawyers. As a group, I do not consider them particularly deep. The one quality, however, that most lawyers possess is that they "think quickly." They may not always give you the right answer, but they will usually give you a quick answer. In litigation and trial work, the lawyers think especially quickly. It's reactive, instinctive: "Objection, hearsay!" These are not deep thoughts, but they are quick thoughts. I couldn't think quickly anymore.

After the deposition experience, I became scared at first, then I just felt sadness. One day, I sat down and journaled a summary of what I had been through up to that point. These words gave me comfort for months:

I think I have figured out what has happened since Thanksgiving. Portions of my brain suffered some defects. These defects have caused memory, thinking, organization

*and visual problems. My brain is slowly getting better. I
don't know if it will get back to "normal." I don't know
what "normal" is.*

*My brain is not me! It's just an organ that "thinks." Not
unlike an ankle, wrist or knee. It's just broken and it needs
time to heal.*

*My brain will do what it can do. I can either remember,
or I can't. I can either figure something out, or I can't. Just
because I can't figure something out or remember something, doesn't mean I'm a bad person. My soul has not been
touched!*

I spent more time with my psychiatrist. He helped me
reduce my stress and wait for my brain to heal. As six
months came and went, I began to doubt that my brain
was going to get any better. I tried to be extremely organized, so that I wouldn't forget things. I took a lot of notes.
I exercised, slept more than eight hours every night and
tried to do one thing at a time. In May, Connie and I had
our second son, Michael. I was physically present, but
did not feel what I had experienced when our first child
had been born two years earlier.

In April and May, I began tiring each day after noon. I
went to work every day and pretended to get things done,
trying to avoid conversations, court hearings and depositions. By the end of April, I contemplated looking for a
new job. I didn't have the nerve to talk to my neurologist
again, because he kept referring back to the stress factor.
He shrugged off the neuropsychologist's tests as having

been given too close to the initial event. Somehow, he believed, my brain had recovered. I grew increasingly angry with him as the months passed.

In July, after nearly two months on my very first anti-anxiety medicine, I stopped by my internist's office and unloaded. He ordered another MRI and some more Prozac. I took him up on both. The MRI showed that my lesions had worsened: The chance of my having a one-time demyelinating disease was out the window. I had MS—no doubt about it.

Looking at the MRIs was both fascinating and depressing. The white spots were the lesions. I guess seeing them was better than just imagining them. They didn't look that bad. My doctor explained that I needed to start giving myself shots of interferon, and that I should return to see him every month. I went home feeling very sad, and Connie and I talked for hours. Because our youngest was two months old, we talked between naps and feedings. She encouraged me to see other doctors, and to take some time off work. I did both.

I was really worried about telling anyone at work, especially the managing partner of the law firm. I felt that once I disclosed the disease, my legal career would be over. The firm would throw me into the street, my insurance would end, I'd be denied disability benefits, I'd have to sell the house and my family would consider me a failure. I started to think that my life insurance was the most valuable asset I had.

On another day in July, I walked into the managing partner's office and shut the door. I began telling him my story. "I thought I was coming down with a head cold. . . ." I really shouldn't have been so shocked and surprised by the compassion he expressed on hearing my story, but I was. I felt better after telling one person about my illness, so then I told a few other partners. They all had the same response: Go home. Don't worry. What can we do? Take care of yourself.

I told everyone that I needed a few months off to "shop" for a new doctor, and get some treatment for this recent exacerbation. In reality, I needed a few months to cope with the diagnosis, my cognitive changes and the "new normal." When I returned to work on Monday to reassign some work, I thought it would be the last day of my fifteen-year legal career. I cried before leaving for the office and, in fact, had a picture taken with my two-year-old son as I left for work in my suit. I was sad because my children, ages two years and two months, would never know their father as a lawyer, a position I had invested years of hard work to achieve. Suddenly, I began to wonder what my children would think of an unemployed father with a progressive neurological disease. I didn't have any answers; I only knew that I couldn't continue working at this time.

I did something that, to me, seemed so drastic, so wrong and so weak. I left the workforce on disability—something I now know happens to the majority of people with cognitive changes from MS. But I didn't know that at the time, and I thought I had failed my family and myself. It's frightening how much of my self-worth was tied up in my job. Leaving work felt like attending my own funeral. I came home from my last day of practicing law even more depressed than when I had left that morning.

Within a few days my sadness deepened. My psychiatrist would later tell me that my anxiety at work was preventing me from feeling my anger and sadness about the diagnosis, and that leaving work allowed me to grieve. I slept and slept. I sat in the backyard, trying to relax and read the paper. Though I was beginning to unwind, I still couldn't read. The words didn't make any sense.

My new neurologist greeted me warmly and asked if he could get me something to drink while we talked. I spent nearly two hours describing every symptom I had experienced in the last year. He asked so many questions. It felt so good to talk to someone who was knowledgeable about "my MS," and who didn't just try to fit my symptoms into a standard MS profile. For the first time in nearly a year, I felt like I wasn't crazy. I came home, hugged my kids and wife, and spent the rest of the summer happily resting and connecting with my family. I also continued to give myself shots, rested and searched for some professional retraining to help with my cognitive deficits.

In January 1999, I started seeing a speech therapist three times a week for cognitive retraining. This woman was a gift from God, an angel sent to change my life for the better. She described my injuries as similar to those of someone who had suffered a head trauma or an electrical injury. Again, I can't tell you how good it made me feel to realize there were other people with the same problems as mine. After spending three months practicing strategies for improving my cognitive functioning, I felt better than I had in years—better than before I had MS.

The therapist explained that my cognitive changes were sudden (like a head trauma), which had made it difficult for me to adjust. She said that many people had the same or worse cognitive problems, but that because they had been born with this level of functioning, they'd had their entire lives to learn how to compensate for the deficits and, consequently, appeared to be normal. When trauma occurs suddenly, as with MS or a car accident, you must work very hard to learn how to compensate for the deficits. The work makes you very tired and very stressed, which, in turn, makes it even harder to function. Sometimes it seems like a vicious circle: feeling the effects of stress, trying to compensate and then suffering from the ensuing fatigue.

Although I became encouraged about my rehabilitation, eight months at home were hard to take. I loved every minute with my children and wife, but I needed to do something more. I started looking in the want ads for a job. I read books and talked to all of my friends about job opportunities. I felt I had the perfect opportunity to begin a new career—one that would not be terribly stressful and would allow me sufficient time with my family.

The problem with spending fifteen years as a trial lawyer is that you don't really acquire very many useful job skills. My typing was slow and I had never sold anything. I was very disorganized, I couldn't drive and anything to do with numbers was a laugh. As the months passed, I began to think I would never return to work, and that depressed me even more.

After Christmas, one of my partners came to my home and we went out for lunch. He was genuinely concerned and asked me many questions. It was hard to explain to him why I was hesitant to return to the full-time practice of law. Whenever I tried to explain my problems with concentration, memory and eyesight, I felt like I was just saying "I'm not smart anymore." At least that's how it felt. I'm not sure he or anyone understands. My poor memory can be remedied by compensatory efforts (Palm Pilots, lists, organization), but as the day progresses toward noon, my ability to process information quickly—to carry on a conversation, say, with more than one person at a time—fades rapidly. My brain feels used up, at least until later in the evening after a few hours of mental rest. To be honest, I do feel "stupid" at times during the day, and I have to remind myself that this feeling will pass.

The very kind partner who visited me for lunch had a wonderful idea, which has felt like another gift from God. I have now returned to my old law firm as the director of professional development for our younger lawyers. Returning to work has had a tremendously positive effect on my health, my self-worth and my relationships. My job is now part of my life, and not my whole life. It serves my needs, and not the other way around. I also spend half a day each week as a volunteer at the local MS chapter, answering phones and questions for people about MS.

The quality of my life has improved these past two years. I feel emotions I never felt before. My relationships with friends and family have deepened. I have better ideas and I'm more organized, so I can put my ideas into action. I listen to my body, and I rest when I'm tired. When I'm hungry, I eat. When I don't know the answer, I say so. When I need more time, I ask for it. I am hugely different from the man I was as a lawyer without MS.

Three cold Chicago winters have passed since my diagnosis. Many of the activities Connie and I once enjoyed are now a part of our history, our past, but we still spend a lot of time in the backyard with our plants. These hardy souls come back every spring to remind me that we are one year closer to a cure.

RICHARD PALMER *lives in the Midwest with his wife, three sons (ages two, three and sixteen) and nephew (age fourteen). He volunteers for the National MS Society and counsels young lawyers on career issues. He enjoys gardening and his saltwater aquarium.*

13

LIVING FROM THE INSIDE OUT

Lisa Desautels

OBSESSION AND LISTENING

As my husband and I sat in the doctor's office hearing her confirm a diagnosis of MS, it was as if the words burst in like a wise guy in a bulging trench coat. Headed straight for us, he reached for his machine gun, pointed in our general direction and fired an enthusiastic round into the air. Then he fled the scene, leaving us with spirits in shambles, a bottomless pit of questions and a knot of fear in my stomach.

His startling intrusion and pernicious presence had only one purpose in mind—to sabotage my spirit, which had been, up until that memorable Friday the 13th, lively and bright. I was thirty-three years old, and all things seemed to be going my way. Just finishing a master's degree, I was finally feeling credible and perceived myself ready to take the professional world by storm. My husband and I were just about to celebrate the first anniversary of a marriage that had been nearly a decade in the making. Although neither of us felt the biological clock ticking too swiftly, we did enjoy musing about the child we might someday have together. Whose nose would he have? Would she be more like him or me?

> THE CHOICE TO COPE AND COPE WELL SEEMS TO WORK, AND I'VE NEVER BEEN SHOWN THAT THE ALTERNATIVE WORKS TO ANYONE'S BENEFIT.

As the walls started caving in, it seemed that the graceful cadence of our new life together was about to give way to discord and imbalance. All around me, I observed family, friends and colleagues reacting in their own ways to what seemed to be a vicious and ill-timed joke; but none of us were laughing.

I became intrigued by the destruction of the human spirit and our questionable capacity to repair it. An obsession with human suffering began to suffocate me like a heavy, wet blanket, under which I saw and felt nothing but a cold, black weight.

Gradually, as my vision adjusted to the darkness, a pattern of metaphors emerged. The result of spirits under siege was always the same: human souls, in every way broken and torn apart. In her heartache hit, country music legend Patsy Cline lamented that she would "fall to pieces" every time her ex walked by. People of all ages talk of relationships breaking up. Alcoholics have spoken of shattered dreams and worlds falling apart. A recent widow might express that she feels as if she's only half a person. Those plagued by emotional instability may be referred to as cracking up, breaking down or as not having it all together. The busy pace of our lives causes us to remark about crumbling under pressure, or feeling scrambled by unwieldy deadlines. The physically challenged, chronically or terminally ill may speak about literally being shaky or unsteady on their feet, and they will admit to a broken spirit, because they believe they can no longer achieve what they once could.

My obsessive thoughts turned to the nursery rhyme in which Humpty Dumpty, that dear old egg, wearing spats and a checkered vest, fell from a wall into pieces without any hope of reassembly. If ever there were a character symbolizing truly shattered dreams, it was Humpty. He had literally cracked up. Poor Humpty Dumpty's spirit was undeniably crushed, and the story reports that neither the power of the king's horses nor his men could rebuild it. I couldn't help questioning such a miserable destiny and wondering, "Well, if they can't, then maybe he can rebuild himself!" "What if," I thought—without intending any disrespect to Mother Goose—"the rhyme ended with our dear old egg picking up his own pieces, pulling them all together and becoming whole again?" And I thought that if my theory could work for a nursery rhyme character, maybe it could work for me. And so, the pattern of my obsession transformed into the notion of rebuilding myself.

It may seem a huge leap from the nursery to the professional world, but my vision of a patched-together egg spirit was confirmed when I looked around at current trends. The pop business culture refers to "self-reinvention," suggesting that in today's fast-paced, high-tech and e-commerce explosion, it has become imperative, more than ever before, for people to learn how to find jobs that will work for them. The popular concern appears to be how we can plug into a rapidly undulating world, and go beyond simply taking a virtual tour of a life characterized by tireless celerity. Without question, an interest in conjoining the mind, body and spirit are at a record high. Everything from aromatherapy to zenith searching in the privacy of your own living room floods our existence, and insists that we keep a spiritual bearing toward living the life celestial.

This theory of self-reinvention sounded great on paper, but the true test would be that of real time spent with my newfound illness. Despite the prolific rhetoric of the New Positive Age, I knew words alone wouldn't completely cut it when it came to the real limitations of my disabled future. The state of the "newly diagnosed" is usually one of overwhelming fear, anxiety and confusion, and I was no exception. The possibility of being old before my time, when I was once content with being known as wise beyond my years, gave me great pause. The thought of soldiering forward to mend my own broken spirit, however appealing, was sadly set aside—at least for the time being.

Almost immediately, I suffered another flare-up and was hospitalized with weakness in my legs. I had the honor of sharing a hospital room with a lovely woman who was approaching ninety years of age with immeasurable grace and sophistication. Marcia loved to read; among her favorites were the works of an early American feminist icon, Charlotte Perkins Gilman, and Britain's meticulous and witty Jane Austen. I instantly liked her and her unspoken resistance to conventional values. We talked about our lives and the events that had brought us each to these beds.

Marcia had taken a tumble and badly cut her leg. The wound was taking longer than usual to heal, and perhaps because of her age, she was fighting infection somewhat ineffectively. She was a survivor, though. She had already outlived her husband by more than two decades, in complete disregard of the statistical odds of spousal dependency and death occurrences. Her courage in his absence was, to me, extraordinary. She talked about her love of life, and how it was the thrill of independence and survival that gave her pleasure and peace of mind. It had become a game, for instance, for her to keep her sons from checking up on her every day.

I told her about my MS, and explained that the slow steroid drip was a treatment for regaining strength in my legs. I was still among the newly diagnosed, and I was unable to talk about my illness without getting emotional. Watching her furrowed brow while I spoke, I apologized for being weepy and explained that I was so terribly frightened about what might happen to me. Marcia looked at me warmly, relaxed her forehead, and said in a slow and concerned manner, "Oh, my dear, has no one ever told you that not one of us knows what lurks around any corner, and more importantly, that fear is paralyzing?"

At first, I was embarrassed at having made it to my early thirties without absorbing such simple and brilliant wisdom. Then I was struck by the youthful light in her face. Her skin seemed smooth, as if its age had suddenly dissolved like lines washed away in the sand. We sat there, silent in our respective mechanical beds, facing one another with a gentle stare: two people, one young and one old, retracing the steps of their lives, assessing where they'd been, how far they'd come and what lay ahead. The moment seemed to last for hours.

The natural inclination for both of us, in that moment, would've been to get up and go to the other for a comforting, supportive embrace. We laughed about the irony of keeping to our beds instead, separate and immobile, like wounded deer in the woods. So, we vowed either to toss handwritten notes skillfully through the air into each other's laps or, more simply, just "chat the time away." When Marcia was ready to leave the hospital after a day or two, I knew that her kind face and wise words would stay with me always—and they truly have.

I had the room and my thoughts to myself after my friend went home. While sitting in the quiet, hooked up to the IV, I watched as the walking world below scurried about like ants around a crust of bread. They whizzed along at a pace that I believed could no longer be mine. How fortunate they all were to experience such freedom of movement! It made me recall the sort of thoughtless way I used to move through life. Rather than being awed and grateful for my everyday abilities to bend, stretch, run, dance, dash, skip and jump without effort, I took it all for granted and believed it was my own entitlement. By this point, I hadn't yet researched multiple sclerosis enough to fully understand the gamut of symptoms that may or may not arise. The fear that had stepped in and slapped a stranglehold on me had convinced me that if I didn't look at this MS thing, it just might go away. Despite efforts to call upon Marcia's infinite wisdom, and fleeting thoughts of resurrecting Humpty Dumpty, I now truly believed I'd never walk again. My spiritual trajectory was downward and inward, with little hope of reversal.

At that moment, a nurse poked her head into my room. She was not one of the nurses who had been tending to me earlier that day by checking vitals or offering lunch. She was a tall, very pretty woman, with eyes that twinkled like a cat's in the night. As she approached, she said in a smooth and serious tone, "Hi, Lisa. I'm Sue. Can I talk to you for a minute?"

"Sure," I said. As she closed the door behind her, I had a sudden sinking feeling. I was frazzled to begin with, fairly hopped up on the steroids and full of jitters; I felt ripe for a full-blown neurosis. Why was she closing the door when it had been open during the last three days of treatments? All I could imagine was the way TV docs, and particularly Marcus Welby, M.D., entered a room to break the fatal news to a patient. I remembered how Welby would walk in while removing a surgical mask, having come straight from an operation or delivering a baby. He'd have a stethoscope firmly in hand, which was then gingerly placed around the back of his neck and draped down along the lapels of his bright white, well-pressed coat or blue scrubs. His head would tilt forward gently, his sullen eyes reaching out to meet the patient's, and he'd say something inane like "I'm afraid I've got some bad news for you, dear."

I must've looked like a stuffed troll with that deep wrinkle across my brow and wild Bakelite eyes so big they'd never close. I mustered the question, "So, is every-thing okay?"

Sue sat down comfortably on what had been Marcia's bed and said kindly, "Oh, everything's fine. I just wanted to share with you that I've had MS for over fifteen years and thought you might like to talk."

A burst of breath and tears came punching out of me as if I'd just been given the Heimlich maneuver—the release of months of anxiety. It was the first time I'd ever reacted so strongly to something without thinking about it first, and it was also the first time I'd ever met another living soul with MS. Now there was one sitting before me, and she wasn't in a wheelchair as I'd imagined. At that moment, she was calm, cool and, to me, the most col-lected, most wonderful human being alive. I had questions but didn't ask them. I had thoughts and feelings but didn't express them. I just listened silently, with a trickle of tears on my face to remind me I was still awake, not dreaming.

Sue spoke of how the first few years are the toughest, because "you've really got to work at getting your head in order." Her tone and manner were so strong and cer-tain, reassuring and realistic, capable and confident with-out being at all arrogant or preachy. She talked about the benefits of getting connected to the MS Society for infor-mation and support. She herself served as a peer-supporter to individuals in need of a compassionate and understanding ear. She shared with me some success stories of other MSers and told me that her own wellness would not have been possible without finding her own truth. She spoke of her life beyond MS, her family and her love of dogs—an interest I shared. Sue made me feel like I didn't have to fade away just because I had this spirit-sucking disease. Then when it was time for her to complete her rounds, she was gone, leaving me with one of the finest messages I'd ever received.

After meeting Sue, I realized I wasn't alone. She had told me that millions of people all over the world are living with MS. That information—especially the words "living with"—would later prove to be a vital part of my recovery and acceptance. I kept thinking about how lively and lovely she was, and that I wanted to be like her, and like Marcia, too: steady and sparked with calm and grace. I don't know what it was that brought the precious miracle of those two women into my life in the same week, but I'm deeply grateful for them. Their impact will long withstand any damage done to my body by demyelination. On that day I began repeating to myself on a daily basis "Find my own truth, find my own truth."

Immersion vs. Denial

The steroids were more or less successful; when I left the hospital, I felt as wild and free as an unleashed animal. As I grew stronger, I wanted life served straight up, without dilution of any kind. There was urgency to everything I did. After enduring MS oddities like vision gone haywire, numbness, weakness, tingling and the sensation of being bound tightly in gauze from waist to toes, I wanted every experience to be a total sensory explosion. My behavior became erratic, odd and extreme. Sometimes I felt as if I was racing off recklessly in a derailed train. I would do things like drive into the sunset on the Massachusetts Turnpike, when the sun's glare was almost blinding, without using the visor or my sunglasses, just to feel the burn of the sun in my eyes. I delighted in dipping my bare hands into the deep snow until they were completely numb, then rushing into the house to run them under scalding hot water until they throbbed, itched and turned purple.

One of the most bizarre of these experiences occurred on a Boston street corner where I'd passed the same homeless person every day on my way to work for nearly two years. My usual pattern was to divert my eyes and involuntarily hold my breath as I passed him and his unbearable stench. This particular morning, however, I looked straight into his yellowed, blood-lined eyes and breathed in as deeply as I could, as if filling my lungs with the freshness of the Rocky Mountains. He looked at me as if I were crazy, and I started thinking that perhaps I was. About the same time, someone close to me had accused me of being in denial, and now I wondered how the hell this could be denial when it felt like total immersion. I thought there had to be an easier way to discovery and acceptance.

I started seeing a counselor as a way of releasing some of the junk building up inside me, like removing a radiator cap from an overheating car. It turned out she was a good listener, and it was comforting knowing she was there; but something was missing, like a mouthful of food lacking flavor when you have a cold. I was beginning to feel talked out with little sense of real resolution. My nights were still sleepless and without comfort of any kind.

The counselor referred me to a psychiatrist, who wrote me a prescription for the perfect drug that would erase all my anxiety and allow me to sleep. All it really erased was my ability to think clearly, offering me little except morning headaches and the feeling I'd been run over by a truck. I gave it up as quickly as I started it. Something powerful was compelling me to hold on tightly to my clarity of thought in a rather desperate way, as if that were the lone life preserver in a terrible shipwreck. When I reflect back upon those less-than-cheery times, I realize that it was all a process I absolutely had to go through.

DISCOVERY AND ACCEPTANCE

I was growing dispirited with the runaway-train activity of my mind, and I longed for the feelings of well-being I'd gained from meeting Marcia and Sue. I found that if I didn't work at cherishing the good times like prized gems, their luster paled, as did my own. Once again, I turned my focus toward the habit of thinking, mostly at night when I should've been sleeping. I thought about Marcia and her frail exterior, and how she was anything but frail or weak on the inside. Her spirit was vibrant and steady, with the calm stillness of an undisturbed lake. Then I thought about Sue and her undeniable courage and strength in the face of our unpredictable illness. On the rare occasions when I had these slices of productive and valuable thought mixed in with the usual fear and anxiety, I'd jot down any shreds that made sense. That way I'd be sure to remember them as I continued my search for illumination.

What came to me from this process of vigorous introspection was the concept of living from the inside out. I decided that living from the inside out is what happens when you activate your soul and your mind first, before considering yourself a victim to the world around you. It means appreciating your impact on life; treasuring your contributions to life rather than believing that all things are simply happening to you without any responsibility of your own; and responding mindfully to life instead of reacting thoughtlessly to it.

I tried to think back to a time when I didn't live reactively, believing that life was there to make me feel fulfilled and happy. Sadly, I went all the way back to when I was a child who thought confessional booths at the church were dressing rooms for the priests. I went back to square one and revisited my Humpty Dumpty theory: the possibility that an individual could have, quite on their own, what it takes to pull a life together, without a magic pill or waiting for the wave of a wand. We've all read about those silent heroes who've run marathons with only one leg, or played beautiful piano despite the brain of a child and never the privilege of a single lesson. The inspirational and remarkable human souls who face and overcome odds daily are all around us. Why not learn from them? Maybe it's all in the way we look at things— and things were looking much brighter to me when filtered from the inside out.

Once I realized the human ability to recognize and alter our perceptions at the very moment we're at our absolute weakest, doors flew open—layer after layer, like one of those mystifying M. C. Escher prints with overlapping, mazelike staircases. What a pleasant discovery to consider the thing sitting inside my head as something other than a gooey mass like the squiggly stuff in a jar in a horror movie. And, although it happens that mine is riddled with these active things the doctors like to call plaques, my mind does not have to be my nemesis. Here was, perhaps, the one thing I could finally learn to control in a body that held more surprises than a busted-up piñata.

I discovered that the only real thing in life any of us can control is the way we react or respond to things; and I realized that I had been living an aberration of untruths for far too long. This nugget of wisdom became, for me, my acceptance. What I chose to do with it remained as unknown as the true origin of the illness pervading my brain and spinal cord.

CLARITY, KNOWLEDGE AND PATIENCE

Duly charged by my new outlook, I proceeded to read all I could about multiple sclerosis, with a watchful eye on the medical profession. I was sure I'd find the one stone unturned, find the cause and the cure and save the world from this insidious disease. My shelves became armed with books about fight or flight, the relaxation response, and taking charge of your chronic illness. I became a student of mind-body practices and set out with determination, and some trepidation, to find the clearing in what appeared to be a wildly dense forest.

In my obsessive quest for knowledge, I felt as if I was trapped inside a snow globe with its weather dial stuck on "blizzard." In the middle of my snow blindness, my father wisely suggested focusing on behavior modification, a subject he'd researched during a fellowship in the behavioral sciences at Stanford University. So, I embarked upon a three-month course to learn some tools and techniques— how to alter unhealthy mind behaviors and how to break entrapping patterns of thinking. What I sought was clarity, meaning and understanding, hoping to turn the fears into challenges. Only then could there be peace, I concluded, and in the ensuing search, ideas appeared to me as readily as morning sunlight unfolding across a clear city skyline.

Through this period of unveiling, I encountered activities like yoga, meditation and creative visualization. The latter, especially, has been a practice I've seized on with passion and deliberateness. The ability to mentally place myself somewhere else has gotten me out of a number of tough spots. Blows brought on by flare-ups full of total despair and zero tolerance, as well as claustrophobia experienced during countless MRIs, have been lessened by the power of willful mind travel. For instance, there's a cliff, hovering three hundred feet above sea level in the narrow Golden Gate of California at Point Bonita. Atop that craggy cliff sits a lighthouse, alone at sea. I've enjoyed the breathtaking view from its watch, and the spray from the waves crashing against the rocky cliff walls. The wind whips by my skin, leaving a moist redness and a lingering coolness, as my lungs fill with the fresh and salted air of the Pacific far below. I've experienced all this, without ever having actually set foot on that cliff, except from within the quiet peace of my mind. With that same ability, I've sat with squinting eyes, dangerously close to the tracks, awaiting the fast clickety-whoosh of the train to whiz by and rattle my ears, tousle my hair and awaken my senses. I've also floated gently in a blissful pool at the base of a waterfall somewhere in Brazil, I think, and the water always exactly suits my temperature-fussy body.

My new learning did not come as easily or quickly as I might have hoped, but like the child whose tongue tires from worrying a loose tooth, I found eventual rewards for my patient efforts. Armed with new knowledge, techniques and the goal of further practice, I now had the strength and clarity to embrace my illness and, ultimately, to live with it instead of against it. While it is with militant refusal that I will fight never to succumb entirely to MS, my conscious and obedient decision toward salvation has been made: adopt the infinite passion of an opera singer, the lively spirit and imagination of a child poet, and the brilliant desire of an artist.

ADJUSTMENT AND FINDING A NEW RHYTHM

At last, there was some hope of finding a way to fit into a world that had been daftly picked up and slammed into pieces against a wall. Things still felt awkward and unshaped, like a coat that was a couple of sizes too big, or like that dizzying, unsettling feeling you get when you awaken in a pitch-black room, before your eyes adjust to the darkness.

Finding a new rhythm by which to move through life is like hearing a song you really like for the first time. You groove to the beat or the melody, whatever it is that strikes you, that moves you, that grabs your attention with the relentless persistence of a metronome. It is something fresh and unknown, but somehow oddly familiar. This is to be your very own new and favorite song. The second time you hear the song, you might try singing along, but you don't really remember all there is to know about it, except that you liked it the first time you heard it. It's still a relatively new experience, a little quirky. Still, it moves you and makes you hum along or tap a finger or maybe even sing along with the wrong lyrics. You feel more acquainted with it, thinking perhaps you'll even buy the compact disc. You do, and you've now heard the same song maybe three or four times and you know the track number by heart. You can follow along with the lyric sheet, and perhaps you've even memorized a few verses. It grows more and more familiar each time you listen. The novelty is wearing off, but what's left behind is the comfort of having found something to make your heart sing, a song that's beginning to feel as familiar as an old, well-worn bathrobe. You're still moved by it, and you have nearly forgotten how awkward you were with it when it was completely strange to you. By the time you've heard the song seven or eight times, you're singing along as smoothly as the bouncing ball that bobbed along the words of those old commercials in the sixties—"safe . . . and . . . rest . . . ful . . . sleep . . . sleep . . . sleep." You've become so familiar with your song that you've even captured the nuances of the vocals and the instruments. You anticipate them. You could even perform your song in a karaoke club, if begged. After hearing your new, favorite song a dozen or so times, you find yourself improvising and making your own rhythm within the actual rhythm of the song. It becomes so much a part of you that it's as if you knew it this well all along.

Whether your new rhythm moves with the fluidity of a gentle piano concerto, the fast-pulsing backbeat of rock 'n' roll, or the thick, slow and soulful outpouring of the blues, it's yours to nurture. It's important to realize that—because of MS—changes may (or may not) develop in your body in a way that'll remind you of a once prepubescent you, awkwardly wearing a body that has to be the misfit of the century. The limitations of an aging body may stroll alongside those changes as unexpectedly as a phone call from an old lover.

The trick now is to have the focus be all about what you can do rather than what you cannot. Perhaps you'll do less, but whatever it is that you do, do it with verve, and remember that living from the inside out is to become more mindful about the giving and contributing rather than the taking and expecting. It is possible to make your new rhythm work, although perhaps a bit differently, just as well as the old one.

At no point along the journey have I deluded myself into thinking the road to self-reinvention would be entirely devoid of bumps; but throughout the course of my quest, I've found enormous comfort and reason to carry along the way. With the support of a loving husband

and parents, friends and the wonderful people at the MS Society, I've learned to dance again in a new way.

Years ago, my favorite nurse spoke to me about the benefits of a peer-support relationship and the power of the two-way communication that can develop. As I've striven to follow Sue's wise lead, I see now, more vividly, what she meant. The experience of being a peer-supporter offers me as much insight and support as I offer to others. In this gratifying role, I talk passionately about mental preparedness, about developing those inner skills before you need them and about allowing yourself time to grieve your losses.

A child once asked me, "Are you okay? Sometimes I see you walking with a cane and sometimes not." I explained that I have a medical problem that comes and goes just like bad weather, and that he needn't be frightened by it. In peer-supporting, we discuss the mental calisthenics that are useful to hone early on and to have on hand later. This way, when the storms come, we're well armed with places to go in our minds where we can batten down the hatches and hold on safely and securely.

LESSONS LEARNED

All of this is not to suggest that I no longer have demons, or that they've all gone off to a convention to haunt the spiritually challenged. My power dreams have me facing fear nose to nose and punching its lights out if

it messes with me. Indeed, fear has become my terma-
gant who, if provoked, comes out of her hideous cave full
of ugliness and rage. She makes bold attempts to chip
away at the hard shell I've created to steel myself from
her wickedness. She tries to undermine my arduous
searches through the corners of my soul, the strides I've
made in leafing through endless pages of my mind's
occasionally unthinkable and gyrating volumes.

My fears disgust and intrigue me, in the same way
we've all sheepishly watched scary movies through timid
and trembling fingers. What terrifies and repels us can
also fascinate and amaze. I know a woman—my older
sister—whose lifestyle of alcohol and drug dependency
horrifies me, yet I find her endless ability to withstand
the harshness of her own self-inflicted pain completely
astonishing. My entire family has made several futile
attempts to save her from herself. It's apparent to me that
one does have to want help. For years, she has sought
solace, not only in a bottle, but in less obvious hiding
places. She frequents tanning salons, but will never be
seen wearing bright colors to show off her darkened skin.
Instead, most days she wears black. What my sister
seems to want is to fade out of sight, much the way an
image does in the rearview mirror as a car slowly drives
away; finally, all we can do is turn and watch.

I often ponder the lifelong lessons learned from this
woman. This kind of learning can be like looking deeply
into an open wound. In a way, I've been fortunate to

stand witness to a wasted life, since much of my memory of her is like a painful photo album, strewn with disheveled and inebriated images in living rooms and emergency rooms—a pictorial lesson in how not to be. She has been my signpost that flashes out, "Seek Alternate Route."

To inhibit the natural progression of learning—painful as our lessons may be—seems to me as criminal as thievery or murder, as unjustifiable as my sister's giving up. There can be comfort in knowing that learning's often invisible friend is hope. The thought of losing that initial phase of discovery and acceptance of my diagnosis is as frightening to me as waking up tomorrow morning without the use of my legs. While it was certainly among the most difficult times of my life, it was also among the most precious and revealing.

My husband once said to me with powerful sensitivity and compassion that, if given the opportunity, he'd trade away the illness that has entered our lives, but he wouldn't want to give up what we've learned from it. The events of the last several years demanded that I reinvent myself; that I redefine and reshape those things that are most important to me; that I reconnect with people who share a similar belief in living from the inside out; that I reposition myself in the larger picture. We mustn't be too alarmed if the larger picture appears altered as old friends, acquaintances and, perhaps, even some family, may no longer fit into the schemata that comprises our new rhythm.

One of the many puzzling things about having MS is that it has made me identify more completely and respectfully with the older generation. There's an unspoken understanding about shared ailments, creaky bones, stiff joints and fatigued limbs. My grandmother, now ninety-three, has become one of my most treasured friends. Perhaps she doesn't know it, but it takes enormous courage to live as long as she has, to watch gracefully as the decades stack up one after the other like playing cards, just waiting to be shuffled and stored away forever. Every time I climb stairs, firmly grasping the railing to pull myself up and along, I follow her steadied pace. Getting up from the bed each morning with bent knees and hips, as I carefully place one foot in front of the other—ever so slowly, with all the stiffness of a heavily starched shirt—out comes a frustrated chuckle, and I fondly think of her.

Having MS showed me that I had been operating at half throttle and had never insisted on appreciating life the way I do now, the way it deserves to be appreciated. My pace was always at the fever pitch of a manic juggler, while the juicy stuff that sits deep beneath the frenzied surface rarely captured my attention. It's a remarkable feeling to suddenly experience being touched by your own sensory-deadened body, moved by your own immobility, to really see with crystal clarity through damaged vision and to listen so attentively with potentially compromised hearing. In some strangely perverse way, this illness has been like an unexpected gift that you cannot return and you must put to good use. We all suffer, have pain and difficult times. From those, no one is exempt. How one deals with a major life change is as personal a choice as having children. For me, the choice to cope and cope well seems to work, and I've never been shown that the alternative works to anyone's benefit.

Part of learning to live from the inside out is recognizing that what's deep inside has to be a healthy soul, as sweet and pleasing a place as the center of a Tootsie Roll pop or some precious gem that hides deep beneath the earth or sea. It's also striving to find what works to allow you to function at optimum efficiency and satisfaction, in a world that you now believe has grown less kind. Indeed, our world changes with all the speed of a caffeinated nanosecond, but that needn't mean we can't find a way to move within it, despite a change in our own personal pace. To find the intellectual force that sparks us, and to build upon that strength of mind to find and create a new rhythm, is a goal worth striving for. The body and soul will ultimately follow suit with equal measures of attention, sensitivity and experimentation. The end result is all the same—nurturing and cultivating our own splendor.

Not long ago, my mother intuitively gave me the children's book *The Little Engine That Could*. It sits on my desk, within easy reach, alongside a figurine of Humpty Dumpty and all the vital books I use to search for answers, definitions or meaning—my sustenance. Not only does my mother's gesture communicate a message of perseverance and self-belief, but it also serves as a warm and loving reminder that we are all still children at our very cores. Peel back the layers of what makes us visibly older and grown-up, dust off the graying images of ourselves as we look into a mirror, and we'll find a simple and glorious innocence bright enough to help us find our way through the darkest of times. Not unlike the decidedly homesick Dorothy, bold and cowardly Lion, most thoughtful Scarecrow and tender Tin Man in *The Wizard of Oz,* what we all desire most is always well within reach—home, courage, sensibility and heart. I suspect that despite periodic and dissonant interruption, the multitudinous noble pursuits we seek in life are quite naturally attainable by each and every one of us. The absolute and comforting glory can be found in knowing that the learning and the believing never cease.

LISA DESAUTELS *has an undergraduate degree in English from the University of Massachusetts at Amherst and a master's degree in English education and language arts from Boston University. She has also completed studies in metaphysical literature at Trinity College in Oxford, England. She has been employed at the Massachusetts Institute of Technology for nine years and is currently a senior research analyst in the Office of Development Research and Systems. She has served as a writing tutor to graduate and undergraduate students and has taught English to non-native adult speakers. She is on the board of* *the Chapter Programs Committee of the National Multiple Sclerosis Society's Central New England Chapter and was named a 1999 Chapter Programs Volunteer of the Year. She has also been a contributing writer for the* MS Connection *newsletter. Lisa's special interests include film, dance and cooking. Among her favorite things are relaxing walks with her husband and dog.*

14

HELPING OTHERS

Charlotte Robinson

After I recovered from my first bout with multiple sclerosis, my parents decided to take a trip to New Zealand. While their decision to travel was not related to my diagnosis, they hoped that I would feel well enough to join them. My mother wanted to walk the famous Milford Trek, and knowing that my father was not much of a hiker, she asked if I'd come along.

My mother and I shared a wonderful adventure, and this marked the beginning of the many times I would test my own limits. After our trip to

231

New Zealand ended, I continued around the world alone with a backpack for six months.

Traveling alone caused me to learn a lot about inner balance. I learned to trust that things would always work out, though sometimes not as I had planned. I felt watched over; many times I ran into travelers whom I had met before, often in places I would never have expected to find them and at the times I needed them most.

> I'VE BECOME MORE POSITIVE IN SPITE OF THE DIFFICULTIES THAT MS BRINGS.

I especially remember when a group of us sat around a table and talked about why we were traveling. Everyone had a different reason. One guy was riding his bike around the world, only because his mother thought he could never complete the task. As for me, I was traveling to prove my MS would not get the best of me.

I had been a geology and outdoor education major in college; the outdoor life had been firmly embedded in my soul long before I was diagnosed with an illness. Although I grew up in New Orleans, I spent many summers during college backpacking and participating in wilderness courses in Denver. At the time of my diagnosis, I was teaching physical education part time at a grade school out West and working on my master's in geology.

Predictably, the diagnosis filled me with all kinds of feelings and emotions. At twenty-six years of age—and an athlete who had completed two triathlons—it was hard to be told that my life would never be the same. But I did find relief in knowing what I was dealing with. I had prayed to God to first help me get a diagnosis—which in itself was a long process—and then to help me deal with whatever I had.

I returned to teaching physical education and felt it only right that I explain to the children why I'd been absent for a few weeks and why I was sitting down so often during the activities. I will never forget an eighth-grade girl who, when I told her class about my disease, broke into tears. Afterward, I pulled her aside and told her everything would be all right. She began to cry again and told me her uncle had MS. "Please don't do what he did," she said. When I asked her what she meant, she told me her uncle had taken his own life. I assured her that this wasn't in my plans, and that I would always do the best I could, given the circumstances.

A few months later, I saw a program on TV about women with breast cancer doing an Outward Bound course. I began to wonder, "Why not people with MS?" My experience had shown me what the outdoors could do for people; I had worked in the outdoor education field for a semester in college and taken juvenile delinquents into the wilderness. During that trip, I'd had a knife pulled on me the first day by a student. Four days later, that same student cried like a baby following a physical challenge he'd met and triumphed over. I realized the impact of such programs in building self-esteem.

I attended the Heuga Center in Colorado to see for myself what this ex-Olympic skier had created for people with MS. After his own diagnosis, Jimmie Heuga had created the center to help others with the disease. His motto— "Look at what you can do, not at what you can't!"—helps individuals look beyond the physical losses they may endure in the course of the disease and focus instead on what remains possible. I decided I had a mission: Having spoken to Jimmie about how he had started his program in exercise education, I decided to carry his ideas a bit further. After you've been through his program, I thought, what's next? How do you test yourself to see if you have reached the limit of what you "can do?"

I spoke to my therapist at the Rocky Mountain MS Center about my idea for an Outward Bound course for people with multiple sclerosis. She thought it was a great plan and offered to help. She even took charge of finding support staff who would be interested in going on the course.

By then, I was no longer working toward my master's in geology, but I still continued to teach. As my contract was being decided for the next school year, the headmaster suggested I take some time off to learn to cope with my disease. Although I thoroughly enjoyed my work, I agreed that I needed some time away from teaching to work at pulling my life together.

And that's when my journey around the world began. I put my plans for an outbound adventure class on hold and took to the open road.

The name and logo of the program I founded—Adventures Within—were inspired by that trip. The logo contains a circle representing the world. At the top of the circle is a mountain scene, representing adventure, and at the bottom is the yin-yang symbol representing balance within oneself.

After those incredible months on the road, I returned to make my dream of Adventures Within a reality. At the Colorado Outward Bound School, I completed a three-day wilderness program, along with nurses, therapists, a doctor and administrators of the Rocky Mountain Multiple Sclerosis Center. It was a very successful program; I believe it made some of the participants better caregivers. I especially remember the time one person felt very uncomfortable about doing an activity. It was a trust exercise and she did not want to participate because of the "unknowns." I reminded her that this is what people with MS live with every day—not knowing what the next day will bring. Jimmie Heuga once said that all people have a beast inside them; that beast is uncertainty, and the people with MS are the lucky ones: We know our uncertainty is MS. We have to learn to live with the beast.

By starting Adventures Within, Inc., a nonprofit organization that provides outdoor activities and confidence-building challenges for individuals with multiple sclerosis, I have created an organization that encourages people to try something new, or to return to doing something they once loved. They just have to be willing to engage in that activity in a different way.

In addition to offering a three-day Outward Bound course, I have expanded the program by working with the Breckenridge Outdoor Education Center—taking people with MS skiing in the winter and offering canoeing, river rafting, ropes courses and horseback riding in the summer. We've had participants from all over the country. One woman had never skied until she signed up for the course. Since then, she and her husband have been back several times. During the last ski course, she was stopped by someone from the ski patrol, who urged her to slow down because she was going too fast. She just looked at him and laughed! Since she uses a wheelchair full-time, she loves the freedom that a bi-ski can give her. (A bi-skier sits in a molded fiberglass shell above two specially designed skis. The two skis give a wide base and help to balance the skier. Any type of disability can be accommodated with adaptive ski equipment, but a bi-ski is the most common for those with paralysis or loss of strength in their legs. It is also an activity that she and her husband can enjoy together since he loves to ski as well.)

During another event that I sponsored, I watched a woman who generally used a wheelchair climb a sixty-foot cliff. She had scratches and bruises all over her legs, but she had never been so proud of her own accomplishments. She even came back to try skiing, and attended another summer program with the Breckenridge Outdoor Education Center.

Adventures Within has allowed many people with MS to test their limits, but it also helps them to decide when they have reached their limits. We try to tailor the activities to each individual, allowing each person to learn what they are capable of doing. Participants also come to realize that many of the activities they previously enjoyed are still within their reach; they just have to be willing to approach them in a different way.

I used to think I was offering so much to those who came to my program, but years of participation have taught me that I learn far more *from* them. I have witnessed incredible strength and courage over the years; I carried that with me when I attempted to climb Mount Kilimanjaro in August 2000 with five other women. The climb was, by far, the hardest thing I've ever done. I suffered from altitude sickness and had difficulty sleeping and eating. Despite the struggle, all six of us reached the summit of Kilimanjaro by 9:30 in the morning on August 30. When we started climbing at 1 A.M., we were treated to one of the most beautiful sights any of us had ever seen: The sky was alive with stars.

There were a few moments when I wondered if I'd make it to the top. One night, when I was doubting myself, I looked down and saw the black cord on my wrist that I'd put on during an Adventures Within course in Colorado a few months before. The other participants and I had stood in a circle and held a long black cord between us, before cutting it to make individual bracelets. I'd worn mine ever since, to be reminded of the strength and courage of the individuals on that course, along with all of the other people I've met through Adventures Within. I cried when I noticed the bracelet during the climb; it gave me the strength to make it the rest of the way.

My adventures to Kilimanjaro brought one of life's lessons home with undeniable clarity: The goals we make for ourselves are accomplished one step at a time.

I consider myself fortunate in that MS has had a limited effect on my physical ability, although it has certainly changed the way I look at life. I have learned to appreciate each and every day. I once heard someone say that having MS was the best thing that had ever happened to him. At the time, I thought he was crazy. But I must admit, I've become more positive in spite of the difficulties that MS brings. One way I do this is by staying focused on the task of helping others with the disease.

Beneath my high school picture in my yearbook I put this quote:

> *I have no yesterdays,*
> *time took them away,*
> *tomorrow may not be,*
> *but I have today. . . .*

My life has come full circle since then, but the quote seems to have more meaning today than it had all those years ago. By staying focused on the present, I appreciate what I "can do" today. I know tomorrow will be here soon enough.

CHARLOTTE ROBINSON *was diagnosed with multiple sclerosis at age twenty-six, at which time she founded Adventures Within, a nonprofit organization that provides outdoor experiences and confidence-building challenges for people with MS. In 2000, Charlotte led a group to the top of Mount Kilimanjaro. You can e-mail her at* www.adventureswithin.org.

15

LIVING WELL

Mark Brennan

As a sailor, I'm bound both to the metaphor and the reality of constantly adjusting and readjusting, catching the wind but moving with intent, responding to changing conditions, enjoying the ride. And responding to the surprises of changed emotions. This involves not being afraid of less than noble emotions, unpleasant thoughts and disturbing reflections.

As I sail, change tack, sail on, always adjusting, a range of super-metaphors are waiting in the wings to claim and define the traveling. As companions, they are often less than comfortable and often presumptuous. The basic three find their expressions under the headings of "self-healing," "heroics" and "hope," which are in turn, presented under the grand conceptualization of "doing battle."

There is a certain condemnation in the mind-over-matter-everyone-can-heal-themselves doctrine. There are physical facts that determine inextricably what you can and can't do, but this does not mean you can't stretch the limits, take risks and surprise yourself, even if there are chemical events that occur in the brain that willpower simply doesn't overcome. If there is any virtue in this doctrine, it lies in training and regularly exercising the mind, just as people must exercise their bodies. Mental health is not a static state. It is, like physical health, a field of existence that we are constantly approaching or moving away from. Acceptance seems to me a better basis for health than domination.

> IT IS HEROIC TO LIVE A GOOD LIFE, AND THIS MAY OR MAY NOT INVOLVE ACHIEVEMENTS OBSERVABLE BY OTHERS.

I find the projection of heroics in some cases nauseating, and in others dangerous. It is a world in which bravery, tenacity and exercise are regarded as laudable, something we should all strive for. It is one of the cruelest cuts to my mind, to be trying to do one's best to do what one can, to be continually isolated by a cult of heroism. One commentator echoed this point when she referred to efforts to redefine the culture of disability, thankfully moving away from a dependent-victim model based on "super-crips," those famous men and women who have "made it." Most times, we have only the publicity reports and selective historical records to go on. "Other people achieve this. What's wrong with you?" Being a real hero is understanding yourself, and responding to that understanding and what you might achieve, in any number of ways physically, emotionally, spiritually. It is not living up to someone else's expectation, or some generalized notion of what constitutes a hero. It is dangerous to strive against your own ability, to be confirmed again and again in your own inadequacy. It is heroic to live a good life, and this may or may not involve achievements observable by others.

This leaves our remaining heading, "hope." It is a commodity that seems to suit observers and how they think sufferers should behave. My criticism of hope is not against the flow of healing juices that envisioning better circumstances might create, or the raw recuperative power generated by commitment. Rather, it is the perpetuation of a dependence on imaginary, outside forces. That dependence often gets in the way of seeing the insignificance of the current state of things, including this life, and being liberated to live beyond hope, as well as beyond fear. These are, after all, alternative expressions of that same dependence on the external. Neither hope nor fear really provides the basis for spiritual and emotional sustenance. As we dance both with suffering and with change, the journey into and then beyond yourself seems to be the one that brings you home. And then you might have the confidence to dance with emptiness. When I cannot achieve this, I revert to the quip made by Pablo Casals on the occasion of his eightieth birthday: "The situation is hopeless . . . now we must take the next step." But this "hope" is a very personal matter, and in the end it is one of the most individual and private of human constructions.

And then, of course, there is the all-encompassing battle that, supposedly, we either win or lose. You can tell by the number of news reports of people who die. That's right: The dead are described as having "lost the battle." My own experience is that life is neither adequately described nor satisfactorily resolved through battle.

When you step off the ship in a foreign port, a clarity is generated by strangeness, a kind of geographically induced existentialism, that you then lose as you settle in. Taking risks has the same effect. To achieve and maintain this clarity, even while doing the washing up at home, on familiar territory, is the reward of practicing mindfulness. This clarity of mind is attainable by sitting, going nowhere while traveling far, seeing the significance of your own insignificance and dedicating your energy to the benefit of others.

In moments of concentrated clarity, it is possible to see all of life as a thin sliver of consciousness wedged into a continuous and immeasurable death, as a precious text placed between seemingly blank endpapers. Yet in their emptiness, they frame existence, its reality, its brilliance and its illusion. Metaphors are all very well, but in the philosophical end, it is how you respond to the details, both of disease and wellness, that matters. Details, and taking the time to see them, small facts, trivial knots and mundane occurrences shape and define the experience of living. The scientist, the detective and the poet share this fascination and respect.

So what are my own details? Should I tell you about the snakes and spiders of pain that inhabit my torso and face, the formless fatigue that appears as nothing, but has the effect of a concrete thing, the bruising spills onto hard surfaces? Or the opportunities to write, talk, promote and support only things worth doing? Or the precious intimacies of friends, lovers, children? Or the sheer satisfaction of sitting, revisiting peace, then carrying it through the day? Even details, simple facts, are the victims of analysis and interpretation. The same detail, like leaving something off the shopping list, can be seen variously as aspects of "my" personality, symptoms of a scarred brain or descriptors of this time of life. All share some common emotional and existential facts. I become overwhelmed to the point of anxiety, panic, disablement when I think I have to respond to too many details, whether they are arranged as a rapid sequence or presented as a field of fragments. I have difficulty accommodating and responding to whole newspapers, TV ads, crowded conversations, meetings, relationships based on head butting and other forms of jostling for advantage. I used to be unable to cope with these very well. Now I don't think that I should have to. I have no capacity, or desire now, to break into communications, to make others see things my way. If I have to respond in a predetermined way and at a pace faster than I can manage, I am disabled and inadequate in the partnership. If I respond, I am inadequate. If I don't respond, I am nothing in the partnership. On the other hand, sitting silently communicates trust and acceptance.

The passionate life doesn't accommodate what might otherwise be seen as healthy compromise. Without MS would it all have been different? Would I have coped better with feeling let down, confronted with my failure as a husband? Could the loss of a marriage of over twenty years really be seen only in terms of a retreat from inadequacy brought on by illness? Or might that illness have been the catalyst for organizational change? I claim no correct analysis, if indeed there is one. Letting analysis substitute for transitory experience is a health hazard. Life is full, immediate, demanding. Living in a state of practiced emptiness is not the vacuous state suggested by the words. In fact, it's a full-time job. Even if I take the details of symptoms and respond with behaviors to alleviate such, I still end up with a healthy formula for living.

Dealing with fatigue requires pace and rest, which leads to empty spaces, absolutely vital for creative enterprise. Spasticity calls for stretching, tai chi, massage, all contributing to a sense of balance. Painful muscles and difficulty moving about suggest weight control. Threat of incontinence requires a nontoxic diet and a well-flushed bladder. Difficulty with too many simultaneous inputs requires focused attention at all times, especially in social situations. Intolerance of cacophonous noise requires avoidance of background, especially electronic, bombardment. All these responses are for me healthy physical, social, psychological, emotional behaviors. Careful attention to these behaviors has allowed me to become the person I like to be, with others and alone.

However, we are not taught to spend time alone, not in a way that engenders growth and strength and good views of ourselves. Solitary confinement, banished to the bedroom, standing in the corner, being sent outside or even farther away, are all forms of punishment. "Alone" is supposed to be lonely, isolating, cause for despair. A person's social self gauges its own worth in terms of what use one is to others, and how one is treated. Being alone, for the most part, pulls this rug right out from under us. Role, status, relationship, possession, location are everything.

But when one becomes unwell, out of the office, not active in the house, in a bed for two with only one, one is forced to live life alone, more inside oneself. For some, this may be an extension of an existing life; for others, an alternative form of what they are used to. For most, it is a complete shock. Yet the possibility is there for the condition to manifest itself as brooding, meditative, reclusive, inspirational. At this time, unless we somehow embrace the singleness of the condition, we run the risk of becoming aliens in our own company. "Well me" finds it difficult to share the bed, the body, life with "sick me." The mirror becomes a weapon spitting out contradiction and destruction, rather than a still pool for reflection.

In the past five years, I have moved toward a peaceful vibrancy that transforms loneliness into solitude, depression into sadness, love into happiness. And my active life is characterized by *not* doing what I am generally known for doing. I am a writer, yet I spend most of my time not writing. I also spend most of my time on my own, and when I spend time with others, it is fresh and special. When we are together, when we are at our best, we choose to remember, rather than simply assume a common memory. We encourage new meanings to wriggle out between us, rather than compete with opposing assertions. We explore possibilities, rather than depend on only personal rights and needs, always miserably undefinable beyond the individual. All this is fantastically creative. And when we make love, this is exactly what we are doing.

I would not say my life is changed, although it so obviously has. I would say I am living more fully aspects of my life that have always existed. I used to live other aspects of my life just as fully. I don't like having MS, but life is still life. The last time I felt close to dying, I spent a good deal of time in my head rowing a beautifully handcrafted boat. I guess I simply wanted to see myself as living. If I had died at that time, I would have done so rowing. But I did not die, and although I promised myself I would not make a career out of my condition, I'd be silly to ignore good material that just fell, so to speak, into my lap. This is not the end, and I have not arrived. I ride the wave of insight afforded by intensity, engagement and commitment, for which the handmaiden is, yes, often crisis, disease, pain. I try not to forget that composure, like disquiet, is transitory. In the meantime, I learn new steps while dancing with emptiness.

My son asked for some advice about what it is that makes life worth living in the face of personal adversity, global injustice, despair. The best I could do was to describe achieving, losing and working back toward a state of mind, such that doing the overfamiliar washing up can be done with the same clarity of mind as stepping off that ship in that foreign port. When traveling far and being still are synonymous. When having MS and not having MS are tantalizingly similar. When wanting to separate water from the shape of its vessel appears both ludicrous and amusing. When clearly life is as a river running.

RIVERS RUN

Sometimes I cannot walk
so I sit
Sometimes I cannot sit
so I lie
Sometimes I cannot stay awake
so I sleep
Sometimes I cannot sleep
so I stay awake
No need to hurry
no need to wait

MARK BRENNAN *has published nine books of poetry,*
including Filtered Light *and* From the Lakes. *He was a*
Senior Academic of Literary and Language Education at
the Charles Sturd University in Wagga Wagga, Australia.
Mark continues to write poetry by the Gippsland Lakes.
His books can be ordered by phone: 011-61-03-5156-0718.

READER/CUSTOMER CARE SURVEY

675705 8862

We care about your opinions. Please take a moment to fill out this Reader Survey card and mail it back to us. As a special **"thank you"** we'll send you exciting news about interesting books and a valuable **Gift Certificate**

Please PRINT using ALL CAPITALS

BA1

First Name

Last Name

MI

Address

City   ST   Zip

Phone # ( ) -   Fax # ( ) -

Email

(1) Gender:
O Female
O Male

(2) Age:
O 13-19   O 40-49
O 20-29   O 50-59
O 30-39   O 60+

(3) Your children's age(s):
Please fill in all that apply.
O 6 or Under   O 15-18
O 7-10   O 19+
O 11-14

(8) Marital Status:
O Married
O Single
O Divorced / Widowed

(9) Was this book:
O Purchased For Yourself?
O Received As a Gift?

(10)How many HCI books have you bought or read?
O 1   O 3
O 2   O 4+

(11) Did this book meet your expectations?
O Yes
O No

(12) How did you find out about this book? *Please fill in ONE.*
O Personal Recommendation
O Store Display
O TV/Radio Program
O Bestseller List
O Website
O Advertisement/Article or Book
O Catalog or Mailing
O Other _____

(13) What FIVE subject areas do you enjoy reading about most? *Rank only FIVE. Choose 1 for your favorite, 2 for second favorite, etc.*

	1	2	3	4	5
Self Development	O	O	O	O	O
Parenting	O	O	O	O	O
Spirituality/Inspiration	O	O	O	O	O
Family and Relationships	O	O	O	O	O
Health and Nutrition	O	O	O	O	O
Recovery	O	O	O	O	O
Business/Professional	O	O	O	O	O
Entertainment	O	O	O	O	O
Sports	O	O	O	O	O
Teen Issues	O	O	O	O	O
Pets	O	O	O	O	O

FOLD HERE

BA1

9396058864

(18) Where do you purchase most of your books?
Please fill in your top TWO choices only.

○ General Bookstore
○ Religious Bookstore
○ Warehouse / Price Club
○ Discount or Other Retail Store
○ Website
○ Book Club / Mail Order

(20) What type(s) of magazines do you SUBSCRIBE to?
Fill in up to FIVE categories.

○ Parenting
○ Sports
○ Fashion
○ Business / Professional
○ World News / Current Events
○ General Entertainment
○ Homemaking, Cooking, Crafts
○ Women's Issues
○ Other (please specify) _____

(25) Are you:
○ A Parent?
○ A Grandparent

16

ADAPTING OUR TALENTS

Inbal Tsur

I can't paint with my hands anymore; instead, I hold the brush in my mouth.

In the days before my illness, painting with my brushes occupied a large part of my time. I painted for pure enjoyment, and I didn't entertain thoughts about showing my work in public or selling my paintings at all.

As early as the age of six, I remember starting art lessons with a private teacher; I still have sculptures and paintings in my room from that period in my life. Over the years, I have used various techniques and experimented with different materials, pastels being a favorite.

As a child, I lived with my parents in Jerusalem. Anyone who knows me will tell you, I have always been strong-willed and very competitive, and I have always said exactly what I think as it enters my mind. If any part of my developing personality would help me to cope with an illness later in life, it would be my independence.

> I HAVE COME TO THE CONCLUSION THAT ART, IN ANY FORM, IS BENEFICIAL TO THE SOUL.

Like all girls and boys in Israel, at the age of eighteen I joined the army and served my two years as a computer programmer in army intelligence. When I left the military, I went straight to a university, which became my second home for the next few years. I began studying mathematics and computer science at Hebrew University in Jerusalem, while working as a freelance computer programmer to support myself. I had always dreamed of becoming an outstanding mathematician, but as I didn't manage to get perfect scores on all my tests, I decided, after a few years, to switch to education. I have to admit that in this field too, although my marks improved, I still did not complete my degree. No doubt, I thought I could afford to take my time. I enjoyed studying, and was in no hurry to go out into the world of work.

Then, in 1986, I was diagnosed with MS. The diagnosis was made quite quickly—maybe too quickly for me to absorb what had happened. I began falling and experienced a loss of balance, and I felt tired and without strength.

The doctor's secretary broke the news to my mother and me. Although she was very kind, I will always remember her as "the bad guy." My mother understood the verdict and what it entailed, and she started to cry. Though I was familiar with the illness, I didn't want to understand what was in store for me. It would take many years for me to internalize the simple statement "MS is for life."

My mother was determined to find a miracle to cure me. For years, she dragged my father and me all over the country to meet every kind of charlatan, trying everything she had heard of, spending a fortune as well as an unending amount of time and energy. Each treatment seemed to work initially, but after a very short period, my situation returned to what it had been before. Finally, my mother gave up.

For the first few years I was still able to lead an independent life. I could drive, and I continued with my studies at the university and my work in computers. I painted, my speech was clear, and I was still fully in control of my body and my life. I carried on with my life as if nothing would change. I was however, becoming easily exhausted; a normal working day was a great effort for me. I began to need a walking stick. I still refused to believe that I needed to change my dreams, or to plan my life any differently.

The illness became more visible, and began to affect me with increasing severity. As my health deteriorated, I found myself terribly lonely at the most difficult time in my life. I began to experience rejection from others who could not cope with the situation. One family friend insisted that I was putting on an act, while another no longer invited me to the annual Independence Day party she always held at her home. Her excuse was she had invited so many people that there was no room for me.

Work had become too much for me (falling in the middle of the street was a clear message to me to take it easier). Having left the university, I felt I no longer belonged within any context of the world, and I was left with nothing to fill the gigantic hole that MS had made in my life.

When I became really helpless, a voluntary organization, Yad Sarah, came into the picture, and I began going to a rehabilitation center. Other helping organizations in Israel provided services as well, lending out medical equipment such as wheelchairs and crutches, and making special vans available for transporting the disabled.

Though there are difficulties within the Israeli health system, the level of medical treatment and aid is advanced. There are two clinics for MS in Israel—one near Tel Aviv and the other at Hadassah Hospital in Jerusalem. Through Hadassah, I began receiving an injectable medication for MS. All three of the injectable drugs are available in Israel. I have also found some benefit from working with community social workers. I am also entitled to receive a sum of money from the Ministry of Social Welfare, but due to some problems within the bureaucracy, I am still waiting to receive it.

For some time, I had a home-health aide living with me. She made my life difficult, treating me as if I were an object. I became thin as a stick. I hardly slept, was neglected and became very depressed. At one point, I actually asked to be taken to a stairway near my home and pushed from the top. I had no will to live. My parents didn't believe the stories I told them about my "helper."

Eventually, this live-in helper was dismissed, and my mother arranged for a kind and caring person named Sarah to live with me. Although Sarah had been warned that my speech was hard to understand, she had no problem at all.

We are now like family to each other, and my life has continued to improve from year to year. My father arranged for a psychiatrist to treat me, and the medication I receive for depression has helped my life considerably. Lately, cooking has become an event in our home. Sarah tries out a new recipe each week, and I am the supreme judge of her experiments.

After regaining my strength and adopting a more positive outlook, I was able to return to the university, and though it was only for a few hours a week and took tremendous physical effort, I enjoyed it immensely. As part of my "return to life," I began to take an interest in how I looked and in the clothes I wore. Slowly I began making new friends who love me for my own sake and accept me as I am.

Today I have more friends than ever before, and this strengthens me every moment of the day. Sometimes I still have fears that I will be alone again, but reality is proving me wrong, and I am beginning to believe that history will not repeat itself, as these are true friends.

I was amazed one day when an art-historian friend came to visit me, saw my paintings on the wall and declared that they were masterpieces. I did not believe her, as I had painted purely for the love of expression and did not fully appreciate my talent. To convince me, this friend brought in a colleague of hers who supported her verdict. The two decided, there and then, that an exhibition of my paintings should be arranged at the prestigious Jerusalem Artists' House.

Several weeks later, I found myself at the opening of my own exhibition, sponsored by the Israeli Painters' and Sculptors' Association. A few months later, I participated in a group exhibition with other new members of the association. Not long after these exhibitions, I had to stop painting, as I could no longer hold a paintbrush or crayon.

Years passed, and the hobby I had loved so much was put aside. I slowly began to realize though, through the other changes that were taking place in my life, that by using different techniques I could still be creative in art.

About a year ago, I began painting with my mouth. My social worker at that time put me in touch with the Association of Foot and Mouth Artists, and after hearing my story, a member of the association came to my house and taught me the basics. I was filled with enthusiasm and excitement, and immediately bought an easel and a special table to enable me to paint comfortably.

My painting is certainly different now. Adjusting to my current abilities, I now paint abstractly, focusing more on color and less on line. I use only watercolors, and enjoy the effect of the paint running down the paper, making interesting shapes as it goes. I need someone sitting next to me, mixing the colors for me and placing the paintbrush in my mouth.

The process is often tiring for me, and sometimes disappointing when the final result doesn't turn out as I had envisioned. Naturally, as with any new technique, a lot of practice is necessary to gain better control. At the beginning, it was far from easy. I felt a lot of frustration—and still do sometimes—but this method of painting provides me with enjoyment and fulfillment, which give me the strength to carry on. I have come to the conclusion that art, in any form, is beneficial to the soul.

Having painting back in my life inspired me. I decided

that I wanted another exhibition, and my paintings were again put on display; this time, many of them were available for sale to the public. I had mixed feelings about this: On the one hand, I was happy knowing I had earned this money myself (after losing my earning capabilities as a result of the MS), and I was pleased that people wanted to buy my paintings. On the other hand, it was very hard to part with them. They represented the many stages of my life: my struggles, my pain, my longing to be engaged in the world.

Another example of adapting my interests to fit my abilities is my use of the computer. In high school and university, I had enjoyed learning about programming and computer science. Later my computer skills were a source of income. For the first few years of my illness, computers played no part in my life. Then I was introduced to Moshe, who became a friend and renewed my interest. He helped to open up many new possibilities. Now that my movement is restricted, the computer is my way of communicating and interacting with the outside world. I have a monitor with a special lens in front to help me see. Surfing the Internet also gives me the chance to "visit" museums throughout the world, and view photographs of both animals and places I might otherwise never see.

The computer has gradually been adapted to fit my needs. In addition to the magnifying lens in front of the monitor, enlarged fonts and specialized control panels help compensate for my poor eyesight. For the past year, I have been trying to master a program called WIVIK that enables one to write using a special switch instead of a keyboard. In this way, I am able to write by myself, and that is important to me, even if it is only to sign my name at the end of a letter.

All in all, my eternal optimism and ever-present sense of humor are what have helped me most to cope with my illness. (Often it is difficult to understand me, not only because of my speech, but also because I am laughing while I'm talking.) I try to make the best out of life. People who don't know me well are surprised, I think, when they meet me and can't detect any bitterness or self-pity. The atmosphere in my home is not in the least sad or morbid. My friends tell me that when they arrive with negative energies accumulated throughout the day, they leave my home in a completely positive mood.

There is hope for a meaningful life with this illness, but the meaning must be found by each person within herself. There is life beyond MS—yes—and even a good one.

INBAL TSUR *lives in Israel with her housemate Sarah and continues to develop her painting skills. Inbal welcomes your comments and correspondence. E-mail her at* inbal-t@internet-zahav.net.

17

STARTING OVER

Debi Allen

When I think of all the dreams I had for myself, when I remember the way I had painted my future, it is difficult sometimes to look at the present day and accept it as my reality. No one ever knows what the future holds, but we draw the paths before us anyway, hoping to bring the heart of our plans to fruition. If anything, multiple sclerosis has taught me to change costumes with greater ease and to confront the daily challenges with strength and courage. Since my diagnosis, I have been to the stage of the Miss Massachusetts Pageant, to the bright lights of network television and to the dusty auditorium where my support group meets. I have been to places I never imagined I would go, confronting losses and challenges with equal strength.

I was born outside of Boston, the second of two children, a colicky bundle of a baby. We grew to be a close family, my parents and brother and I, our lives defined by church, community and family. I was very active as a child, involved in sports and engaged in life. I had a stack of big dreams rolling around in my blonde-haired and blue-eyed head.

> WHEN AN MS EPISODE MARCHES IN, IT OFTEN TAKES YOU AND DRAGS YOU FAR FROM HOME. . . . AND NOTHING BUT HARD WORK AND DETERMINATION CAN BRING YOU BACK.

The first signs of physical illness became evident in fifth grade. I was thought to be a hypochondriac at the time, as I was frequently sick. I was eventually diagnosed with some learning disabilities, and it wasn't much later that I developed problems with incontinence, shaking and muscle spasms. I thought nothing of these symptoms, though, given my age, thinking they must happen to everyone.

When I reached high school, I began to experience severe depression, followed by some hearing loss, but once again, I found a convenient excuse: Perhaps my first broken heart was the cause. When I finally went to our family doctor, I was told that my symptoms were "all in my head." I was put on antidepressants and given a host of other medications, but they didn't help at all. I knew that I was ill, yet no one was taking me seriously.

I suppose being young didn't allow me to have much of a voice. Convinced I had a brain tumor, and very depressed, I decided taking my life would be a better alternative. When I was admitted to a psychiatric treatment unit, I too began to question my sanity.

I managed to graduate from high school, but I wasn't quite sure what I wanted to do with my life. Wanting to take some time for myself, I decided to take a year off from studying. I worked at various odd jobs and discovered a love for dancing, aerobics and water-skiing in my spare time.

When I was ready for college, I majored in liberal arts and human services, but my dance classes at school were what I loved the most. Dancing filled me with joy, and renewed my passion for life. Yet deep inside, I sensed there was something wrong with my body; the symptoms I had been experiencing for almost ten years continued to plague me, and it wasn't long before the depression returned. Once again, thoughts of taking my own life overwhelmed me. It was back to the antidepressant drugs and psychiatric hospitals. I was convinced there was something physically wrong with me, but I seemed to be the only one who knew. Living in denial and uncertainty for so long was beginning to take its toll.

A part of me yearned to create a life for myself; I wanted to make my way in the world. Each time my physical or mental health dealt me a blow, I'd get back up and dust myself off. Once again, I returned to school, picking a major I felt I could handle this time around: dental assisting. I picked up a part-time job as a dental receptionist, and upon graduating was offered a job. I found a roommate and moved out of my parents' home, happy to be on my own. Maybe things were going to be all right after all.

However, my MS diagnosis wasn't far away. While at work one day, my right foot fell asleep; as the day passed, the numbness moved up to my right hip. I figured it was just a pinched nerve that would take some time to heal. So I carried on, as I had taught myself to do, numb from head to toe.

The morning I woke up to find my head spinning and my vision blurred marked the beginning of the end: the end of denial, the end of my silent questioning. I called my parents to describe this new round of symptoms and, just like many times before, we set off for the hospital. I was treated for an inner ear infection and then released, still nauseous and very dizzy, and no closer to the truth than I was in fifth grade.

Fresh out of options, we made an appointment with my primary-care physician, who recommended I see a neurologist. After undergoing a round of tests, I sat with my parents and brother in the neurologist's office to hear the final diagnosis.

I'll never forget that day—September 15, 1995. The neurologist started off my appointment by showing us the MRI films, where a dozen white and black spots seemed to scatter across the picture of my brain. When I asked what they were, the doctor asked me to guess.

"Blood clots?" I asked out loud. "Aneurysms? Tumors?"

My mother finally came up with the right answer; the doctor at the hospital had mentioned MS as a possible diagnosis during one of my previous visits to the emergency room. Being young and naïve, I decided I was one of "Jerry's kids" now, but the neurologist explained that I had multiple sclerosis, and not muscular dystrophy. He went on to explain, very vaguely, what MS was and what treatments were available. He said there was no cure. He also told me I "just had bad luck" and gave me a kit for interferon therapy. I left with the kit and a vague description of what I had, with a follow-up appointment set for three weeks away.

I wasn't feeling any better when I went back to see him, so he wrote a prescription for oral steroids and spoke to me again about my "bad luck." My family and I decided it was time to get a second opinion. If any amount of bad luck was involved in this situation, I decided, it had come in finding this neurologist.

Almost immediately, I found a new neurologist who reviewed my records and performed a neurological exam. He decided to send me to a prominent MS clinic in Boston, though I'd have to wait three weeks for an appointment.

Three weeks, it turned out, was too long to wait. One night while making dinner with my roommate, I decided to lie down for a bit, as I was suffering from a headache. When I awoke, the right side of my jaw hurt. The numbness was gone, but severe pain had taken its place. I couldn't open my mouth, because my jaw had locked shut. It felt as if my whole body was shutting down. Just when it seemed like it couldn't get worse, I started getting sick to my stomach, which was difficult because I could hardly open my jaw. With my appointment at the MS clinic nearly twelve hours away, each minute seemed to bring on a new symptom. I felt weak and started falling on my way to the bathroom. I realized I wasn't going to be able to hang in there much longer.

With the world spinning around me, my roommate managed to get me into the car, which was difficult, because I could no longer walk. Talking, seeing straight or doing anything that required strength seemed impossible.

There was really nothing funny about this situation, but sometimes when we look back, we can find a bit of humor in the chaos. On the way to the hospital, we got a flat tire. My roommate and I looked at each other knowingly; this was just our luck. It seems whenever we do something together, it always turns into an adventure. On top of it all, in the commotion of trying to repair the tire, she locked the keys inside the car. We must have been a sight, parked on the side of the highway—my roommate trying to get the keys by climbing through the backseat.

With my head extended out the window as I continued to get sick, my blonde hair blowing in the wind, I was happy to get underway again, to a place where I could finally get some treatment. Before arriving at the hospital, I noticed I had lost the hearing in one of my ears.

I spent the next three months in a hospital. The doctors weren't sure how much, if any, of my normal functioning would return. I was afraid that I would never be the same, and I cried myself to sleep every night. Eventually, I improved and was transferred to a rehabilitation hospital, where I learned how to live my life all over again.

Little by little, with the help of pool therapy, I began to get my strength back. The resistance of the water was a big challenge to overcome, but it was there in the pool that I could actually stand and walk a bit on my own. Then came the day I could walk on land with a walker, then with Canadian crutches, then totally on my own with a little help from the walls. It felt so good to be on my feet again; I wanted to run.

My rehabilitation was sometimes painful, often frustrating and always exhausting, but it was all worth it. I never knew just how much determination and stubbornness I had in me. I wondered sometimes if it was my fear that was motivating me, until I realized I was never on my own. I felt that God was right there with me all along.

During my three-month stay in the rehabilitation center, I collected donations for the MS Walk slated to take place in April. A few weeks before the walk, I was released from the center under full-time care. I moved into my parents' house again, and I was allowed to go back to my apartment on the weekends. The first time I went home to my apartment, two friends carried me up the stairs; I was greeted with a surprise party they had arranged with all my friends waiting to welcome me home.

When the MS Walk took place two weeks later, I brought my wheelchair in case I got tired. It had only been fourteen days since I had left the hospital. I ended up needing it—though, I am proud to say, only for the last couple of miles. My team placed third for collecting donations and we received a bronze plaque.

I was on the long road to acceptance. I began to search for a support group, but it took a while before I found one that was right for me. Through a friend's recommendation, I also found a therapist who specialized in MS and chronic illness. This therapist was wonderful; he helped me go through all the stages of grieving, which is important to do when you are losing a part of yourself.

When an MS episode marches in, it often takes you and drags you far from home. When you wake up, you are miles from your own pillow, and nothing but hard work and determination can bring you back to your own clapboard house with the shuttered windows. Despite my own reluctance to walk that road again, I had another relapse, almost one year to the day after my last one. I quickly understood who was boss—and it wasn't me. My doctors decided that chemotherapy would be the best route this time, since they had a good idea of what they were up against now. After I began the chemotherapy, I was marched back to the rehabilitation center; once again, I struggled to regain everything that multiple sclerosis was trying to steal away. Fortunately, I fared better than I had the last time, though I was still unable to run and had continued problems with balance and coordination—a difficult situation for a former dancer.

In retrospect, it seems odd that I would choose to become a model and actress next, given my symptoms, but that's exactly what I decided to do. It had been my childhood dream. I had a bit of trouble with the runway when modeling in high heels, and often the spasms and tremors in my legs didn't allow me to walk with much grace. Nonetheless, I finished modeling school and found some work doing promotional modeling jobs, some of which required me to go on the road. I loved every minute of it. I appeared in a commercial for Bud Light and on a billboard for Rhode Island Transportation.

I guess I was on a roll, because one evening, while watching the Miss USA Pageant, I called the number that appeared at the end of the show for anyone who had an interest in competing in the pageant. I dialed the number, and, eventually, I entered a competition in Boston for the Miss Massachusetts/USA pageant and was accepted right away.

So began the process of getting sponsors, an interviewing outfit, evening gown, bathing suit and shoes for each event. When the competition began, I was ready, despite having to wear a partial wig; I had lost a lot of hair during my chemotherapy treatments and had also lost a lot of weight.

In the end, I didn't win, but I felt like a winner anyway. I was very proud that I had made it so far, despite all of the obstacles. It was an experience I never dreamed of having—and will never forget.

The pageant opened many other doors for me. Since then, I have appeared in many news articles and other publications pertaining to MS. I also became a peer support counselor with the National Multiple Sclerosis Society, so I can reach out and help others with the disease; I want other people to realize that if I can swing back from adversity, even when the doctors said it wasn't possible, they can too.

Last year, I was fortunate to be chosen to appear on the *Montel Williams* show. I had written him a letter when he was diagnosed with MS, as we both receive care at the same MS clinic, and I wanted him to know that he was in good hands. A few days later, I received a letter from him asking me to come to New York, so I could try out for a segment on the topic of multiple sclerosis for his daily television talk show.

After four weeks of phone calls and discussions, I learned that I was chosen to be one of four women to join him on the show. I'd be lying if I told you I wasn't excited! I took my mom to New York with me, and after we were brought to our hotel, an assistant whisked us off to Montel's offices. They wanted to shoot some footage of me on the streets of New York. Montel and his staff couldn't have been nicer, and together, we pulled off an interesting and informative show on MS.

One of the best benefits of being on Montel's show was meeting another guest. Kate was diagnosed with MS when she was only nine years old; she also has epilepsy. Yet she is one of the most positive people I know. I left New York feeling blessed, and Kate is now like a little sister to me. Although she lives in Oklahoma, we continue to talk and visit each other. I feel like I'm part of her family.

I have been in remission for almost two years now, though I continue to struggle each day with my symptoms. Some days are better than others. My life has been a long and sometimes frustrating road, but I do have a deeper understanding now. I have become a much stronger person and can handle more than I ever imagined.

I didn't choose to have MS, but somewhere along the way, I learned to accept it and make the most of it. I am thankful for the experiences I've had since my diagnosis; they have helped to keep me believing in myself. I now know that we are never too old, never too sick, never too far down the road to dream.

DEBI ALLEN *works as a volunteer peer support counselor for the National Multiple Sclerosis Society. She lives in Massachusetts with her two cats. Debi welcomes e-mail at* Debi0416@aol.com.

In Support of
Multiple Sclerosis

In support of multiple sclerosis research and efforts, a portion of the proceeds of the sale from each book will go to the following organizations.

The Montel Williams MS Foundation

When talk show host and actor Montel Williams was diagnosed with MS in 1999, he made a pledge to use his celebrity to find a cure. True to his word, he established The Montel Williams MS Foundation to further the scientific study of MS.

The goal of The Montel Williams MS Foundation is to provide financial assistance to select organizations and institutions conducting research, to raise national awareness and to educate the public. Currently, 100 percent of the donations received go directly to funding research to find a cure for MS. The foundation makes grants to three research centers: The Brigham and Women's Hospital at Massachusetts General Hospital of Harvard University, a comprehensive care and research center; The Nancy Davis Center Without Walls, a collaboration of leading scientists at top hospitals and universities; and The Karolinska Nobel Institute in Stockholm, Sweden, a trailblazer conducting groundbreaking research.

Contact: The Montel Williams MS Foundation, 331 West 57th Street, Suite 420, New York, NY 10019.

MSWORLD

MSWorld is a comprehensive online support network for people living with multiple sclerosis. Contact: MSWorld at *www.msworld.org*.

RECOMMENDED
RESOURCES

EDUCATIONAL PROGRAMS

The Multiple Sclerosis Association of America:
800-LEARN-MS. 706 Haddonfield Road,
Cherry Hill, NJ 08002. *www.MSAA.com*.
Provides information on patient-care services,
symptom management and living day to day
with MS, offers a toll-free telephone hotline
and a program to help modify homes for
people with MS.

The Multiple Sclerosis Foundation: 800-441-
7055. 6350 North Andrews Avenue, Fort
Lauderdale, FL 33309. *www.msfacts.org*.
Provides information and education to people
with multiple sclerosis. Support line open from
9:00 A.M. to 7:00 P.M., Monday through Friday,
offering free peer counseling over the phone.
Publishes a free quarterly news magazine
focusing on traditional and alternative therapies, and maintains a lending library: Upon
request, will send a book from its library and
provide return postage. A home health-care
division, and a referral service are available also.

275

National Multiple Sclerosis Society: 800-Fight-MS. 733 Third Avenue, New York, NY 10017. *www.info@nmms.org*. A comprehensive support program offering information and education to people with MS and their families.

OTHER INFORMATION SOURCES

Avonex® Support Line: 800-456-2255. *www.biogen.com*. Sponsored by Biogen, provides information about the drug Avonex® and related training materials.

Betaseron® Champions of Courage Program: 800-788-1467. *www.championsofcourage.org*. Recognizes the accomplishments of people with MS, and provides grants to help people with MS achieve their goals and inspire others. To apply for a grant, individuals must be taking the MS medication Betaseron®, describe their community involvement and outline how they will use a grant to inspire others. Contact the program for an application. Applications are reviewed three times per year: February, June, October.

Consortium of Multiple Sclerosis Centers (CMSC): 201-837-0727. c/o Gimbel MS Center, Holy Name Hospital, 718 Teaneck Road, Teaneck, NJ 07666. Made up of numerous MS centers throughout the United States and Canada. Disseminates information to clinicians, increases resources and advances the standard of care for multiple sclerosis.

The Heuga Center: 800-367-3101. P.O. Box 491, Edwards, CO 81632. *Info@heuga.org, www.heuga.org*. Offers a series of multidisciplinary programs for people with MS and diabetes, focusing on a "can do" approach to disease management. Strives to empower participants to live healthy, active, fulfilling lives.

Learning How—OpportunityPlus: 704-376-4735. P.O. Box 35481, Charlotte, NC 28235. Seeks to build self-esteem and confidence